Wellness
Optimal Health and Longevity

Fitness, Health & Nutrition was created by Rebus, Inc. and published by Time-Life Books.

REBUS, INC.

Publisher: RODNEY FRIEDMAN
Editorial Director: CHARLES L. MEE JR.
Series Editor: THOMAS DICKEY

Editor: WILLIAM DUNNETT
Text Editor: LINDA EPSTEIN
Associate Editor: MARY CROWLEY
Chief of Research: CARNEY W. MIMMS III
Copy Editor: ROBERT HERNANDEZ
Contributing Editors: JAN FREEMAN, JANE SCHECHTER

Art Director: JUDITH HENRY
Project Art Director: FRANCINE KASS
Contributing Photographer: ANDREW ECCLES

Time-Life Books Inc. is a wholly owned subsidiary of

TIME INCORPORATED

Editor-in-Chief: JASON McMANUS
Chairman and Chief Executive Officer: J. RICHARD MUNRO
President and Chief Operating Officer: N.J. NICHOLAS JR.
Editorial Director: RICHARD B. STOLLEY

THE TIME INC. BOOK COMPANY

President and Chief Executive Officer: KELSO F. SUTTON
President Time Inc. Books Direct: CHRISTOPHER T. LINEN

TIME-LIFE BOOKS INC.

Editor: GEORGE CONSTABLE

Executive Editor: ELLEN PHILLIPS
Director of Design: LOUIS KLEIN
Director of Editorial Resources: PHYLLIS K. WISE
Editorial Board: RUSSELL B. ADAMS JR., DALE M. BROWN,
ROBERTA CONLAN, THOMAS H. FLAHERTY, LEE HASSIG,
JIM HICKS, DONIA ANN STEELE, ROSALIND STUBENBERG
Director of Photography and Research: JOHN CONRAD
WEISER

President: JOHN M. FAHEY JR.
Senior Vice Presidents: ROBERT M. DESENA, JAMES L.
MERCER, PAUL R. STEWART, JOSEPH J. WARD
Vice Presidents: STEPHEN L. BAIR, STEPHEN L.
GOLDSTEIN, JUANITA T. JAMES, ANDREW P.
KAPLAN, CAROL KAPLAN, SUSAN J. MARUYAMA,
ROBERT H. SMITH
Supervisor of Quality Control: JAMES KING
Publisher: JOSEPH J. WARD

FITNESS, HEALTH & NUTRITION

Wellness

Optimal Health and Longevity

Time-Life Books, Alexandria, Virginia

CONSULTANTS FOR THIS BOOK

James R. Brown, M.D., M.P.H., is the Director of the University Health Service at the University of California at Berkeley. A former Peace Corps physician, he is board certified in pediatrics and preventive medicine. He is also a member of the editorial board of the *University of California, Berkeley Wellness Letter.*

Karen Hughes, M.P.H., is the Director for Alcohol Policy Initiatives Project of the Trauma Foundation in San Francisco, California, which provides training and education related to alcohol and injury prevention for community groups. She also edits the *Bulletin on Alcohol Policy.*

Steven Lamm, M.D., is a Clinical Assistant Professor of Internal Medicine and former Director of Medical Student Health Services at the New York University School of Medicine. He maintains a private practice in internal medicine and is the Medical Director of Life Extension, Inc., which is a health-maintenance organization.

David T. Lowenthal, M.D., Ph.D., is a Professor of Medicine, Pharmacology, and Exercise Science at the University of Florida College of Medicine, Gainesville, and Director of the Geriatric Research, Education, and Clinical Center of the Gainesville Veterans Administration Medical Center. A competitive runner, he serves as the chief medical officer for the United States team to the Maccabiah and the Pan American Games, and is vice president of the American Medical Athletic Association.

Allan J. Ryan, M.D., is the editor-in-chief of *Fitness in Business* and the former editor-in-chief of *The Physician and Sportsmedicine* and *Postgraduate Medicine.* He is the president of the National Association of Governors' Councils on Physical Fitness and Sports, a former president of the American College of Sports Medicine and a member of many sports medicine and orthopedic organizations.

Myron Winick, M.D., is the R.R. Williams Professor of Nutrition, Professor of Pediatrics, Director of the Institute of Human Nutrition, Genetics and Human Development at Columbia University College of Physicians and Surgeons. He has served on the Food and Nutrition Board of the National Academy of Sciences and is the author of many books, including *Your Personalized Health Profile.*

For information about any Time-Life book please call 1-800-621-7026, or write:
Reader Information
Time-Life Customer Service
P.O. Box C-32068
Richmond, Virginia 23261-2068

TIME-LIFE is a trademark of Time Incorporated U.S.A.

Library of Congress Cataloging-in-Publication Data
Wellness: optimal health and longevity.
    (Fitness, health & nutrition; vol. 20)
    Includes bibliographical references.
    1. Health. 2. Self-care, Health. 3.
Longevity. I. Time-Life Books. II. Series:
Fitness, health, and nutrition.
RA776.W44 1989 613   89-20178
ISBN 0-8094-6142-0
ISBN 0-8094-6143-9 (lib. bdg.)

This book is not intended as a substitute for the advice of a physician. Readers who have or suspect they may have specific medical problems should consult a physician about any suggestions made in this book.

CONTENTS

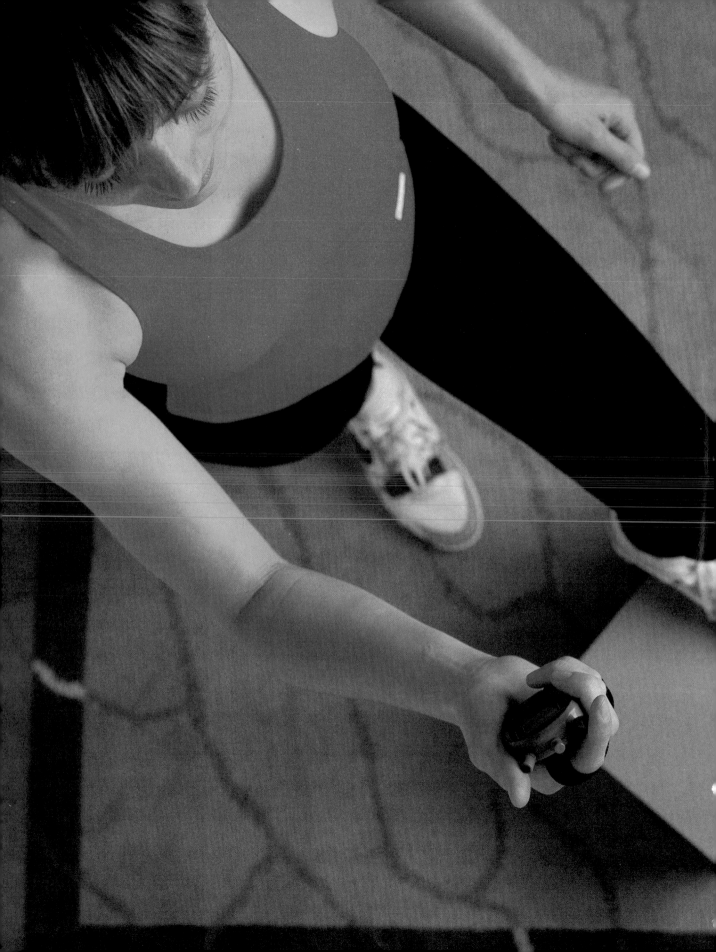

CHAPTER ONE

Assessing Your Health

An introduction to wellness

T raditionally, good health has been thought of as simply the absence of illness, and preserving health has, for the most part, been entrusted to doctors and the medical establishment. Recently, however, a new concept of health care has been evolving — one that involves taking a more active approach to improving and maintaining your overall condition. The concept is called wellness, and it refers to a way of living, not a specific mode of treatment or formula for good health.

The central tenet of wellness is that advances in medicine, while certainly beneficial, are not sufficient to protect and enhance your health. Rather, good health depends upon a wide spectrum of life-style habits that range from diet and exercise to managing stress to safety precautions. Wellness, in effect, is about the choices you make that affect your health, some of them on a daily basis. This book is a guide to help you choose wisely. By using the information in it, you gain two incomparable benefits: You can live longer and also increase the quality of your life, achieving an optimal state of physical and mental well-being.

Wellness does not mean that doctors and medical care are to be avoided: It is not "alternative" medicine. Well-trained medical personnel can help you cope with and alleviate many health problems; moreover, part of staying well involves having routine checkups, immunizations and taking advantage of other techniques that can help reduce your chances of becoming ill. Nevertheless, a great deal of effort within the medical community is directed toward helping people get well after they have become ill. Yet, over the past decade, more and more research has been done to indicate that numerous health problems are preventable.

Although wellness is a relatively new idea, it has already had a significant impact on health care in the United States. According to a recent report issued by the U. S. Department of Health and Human Services, the overall mortality rate from heart disease dropped 31 percent between 1970 and 1986. The report also noted that infant mortality — a common measure of national health — declined 2 percent from 1985 to 1986. More effective treatment is certainly a factor in reducing these figures, but experts attribute the major cause to a general improvement in people's health and a reduction of many risk factors of heart disease, such as giving up smoking and improving diet. Another factor may be that more people are exercising.

Unfortunately, not everyone is benefitting from the growing knowledge about wellness. While the average white American's life span is increasing, the life spans of blacks are actually decreasing. In addition, the mortality rate from lung cancer among all segments of the population is rising significantly; for women, the incidence of lung cancer is especially alarming, since it has nearly doubled between 1970 and 1986. Fortunately health warnings about the dangers of smoking appear to be reaching the public — the incidence of teen-aged female smokers dropped from 22 percent in 1977 to 15 percent in 1985. However, the resulting reduction in lung cancer mortalities will probably not be evident for 30 years.

One of the factors apparently responsible for better health is self-awareness. Studies show that the more people know about wellness, the more likely it is that they will be healthy. The Stanford Three-Community Study mounted a two-year bilingual mass-media health campaign in two communities; a third community, which was used as the control, did not receive health information. At the end of the campaign, researchers found that both men and women who were informed reported dietary cholesterol reductions of 23 to 34 percent. In addition, their saturated fat intake declined by 25 to 30 percent, and their blood cholesterol levels improved. Members of the control community, meanwhile, experienced an increase in body weight.

The Stanford Three-Community Study further revealed that people of lower socioeconomic status may be most at risk of coronary artery disease, lung cancer and other illnesses that limit longevity, but they stand to benefit the most from improved knowledge about health. Although Spanish-speaking participants reported higher dietary cholesterol and saturated fat than English-speaking subjects at the beginning of the study, they indicated having significantly greater health improvements at the end.

Learning how to integrate healthy practices into your daily routine is a natural complement to an active lifestyle. Studies illustrate that the more physically active people are, the less likely it is that they will develop a wide range of illnesses, including coronary artery disease, stroke, hypertension, diabetes, infectious diseases, osteoporosis and osteoarthritis. One study showed that women who began exercising during their youth and continued an active lifestyle throughout their lives experienced a lower incidence of nearly all forms of cancer than their sedentary peers. A study of nearly 17,000 Harvard graduates revealed that people who exercise regularly and participate in vigorous sports are likely to outlive their sedentary classmates by several years. Indeed, the average increase in longevity that an active lifestyle imparts would be about equal to a life span extension for the average person if all forms of cancer were miraculously eradicated.

Attaining and maintaining wellness involves three steps. First, you must assess your current health and determine which risk factors might predispose you to a particular disease. Then you must evaluate those risk factors and find out how you can eliminate them or at least minimize their effects. Finally, you should strive to improve your overall health and fitness through diet, regular exercise, hygiene, and periodic medical checkups and self-examinations.

The purpose of this chapter is to increase your awareness about your current state of health. The true-or-false quiz on pages 10 and 11 tests your specific knowledge in a number of health-related subjects. This test gives you an introduction to the concept of wellness. The test on pages 12 and 13, Your Medical Age, reveals how you apply your knowledge about health to your own life, and delves into your family history and lifestyle factors that may predispose you to illness. Your score on this test may be higher or lower than your actual age, depending on those factors. The Health-Risk-Assessment Questionnaire on pages 14 to 19 shows you the specific areas of health that may need improvement in order to reduce your risk factors. The Step Test on pages 20 and 21 measures how well your heart recovers from exercise and assesses your aerobic fitness.

Since health is a continuing process rather than a static condition, your aerobic fitness, risk profile and medical age may change over time. Therefore, it is a good idea to take these tests every few months. Your aerobic fitness, for instance, will probably improve significantly once you have implemented a regular exercise program, such as the one outlined on page 85. If you were previously sedentary, your medical age will decrease by two years even if you do nothing else to improve your health. By implementing other health habits outlined in this book, you can lower it even further.

S *tudies show that becoming aware of health risks and benefits can even improve the lives of people with incurable diseases. Arthritis patients were given a course on their condition and its relationship to stress, nutrition and exercise. When compared to a control group of similar patients who were not informed, the experimental group had 25 percent less pain, a 20 percent decrease in swollen joints, a 14 percent reduction in disability, an 18 percent drop in depression and a 20 percent increase in their sense of personal competence.*

True or False

The following true-or-false statements are designed to test your knowledge in some specific areas of health and to clarify some widely believed myths about these topics. There is no score, but some of the answers may surprise you.

1 You can reduce the health risks of tobacco smoking if you switch from cigarettes to pipes or cigars.

False. Pipe and cigar smokers are at risk of cancer even if they never smoked cigarettes. And if you are a former cigarette smoker who has switched to pipes and cigars, your risk is greater.

Although most pipe and cigar smokers do not inhale smoke, and are therefore at lower risk for lung cancer than cigarette smokers, they are likely candidates for cancer of the lips and mouth. But former cigarette smokers who switch to pipes and cigars not only tend to smoke more, they are likely to inhale the harsh pipe and cigar smoke without thinking. Studies show that cigarette smokers who use pipes and cigars continue to risk lung cancer as well as heart attacks to the same extent as when they smoked cigarettes.

2 Butter will soothe the pain of a minor burn.

False. Butter is not only ineffective for relieving pain, it may contaminate the wound if a blister forms and breaks. In addition, anything that you put on a burn will eventually have to be washed off, causing more pain and irritation.

Cold water is the most effective treatment for first-degree burns, in which only the outer layer of skin is injured, because it not only relieves pain but cleanses the wound as well. Immerse the burn in cold — but not iced — water for 15 minutes. For more severe second- and third-degree burns, in which the skin is blistered or even charred, cover the area with sterile gauze and get professional help.

3 Even if you have had a tetanus shot, you may not be immune.

True. Tetanus immunization lasts for about 10 years. Also known as lockjaw, tetanus is a bacterial infection that results in muscle paralysis and sometimes death. Because immunization is so widespread, tetanus infections are relatively rare. However, over 70 percent of all cases reported in 1986 occurred in people over 50. The Centers for Disease Control warns that most adults over 60 are not adequately immunized. Booster shots should be given every 10 years. And just to be safe, you should also have a booster shot if you get a puncture or a deep, ragged wound.

4 Cottage cheese is a good source of calcium.

False. You would have to eat about 13 four-ounce servings of cottage cheese to meet the recommended dietary allowance for calcium. While the RDA for most people is 800 milligrams, a serving of cottage cheese contains only 60 to 70 milligrams. (Since it is recommended that postmenopausal women consume 1,200 to 1,500 milligrams of calcium, they would have to eat at least 20 servings of cottage cheese a day.)

Low-fat milk and yogurt are excellent sources of calcium, both supplying 300 to 400 milligrams per cup. Other cheeses, too, are better sources of calcium than cottage cheese, although most are high in fat.

5 Older drivers are safer drivers.

False. Drivers over 65 tend to have a worse accident record than any other age group except those under 25. Although people over 65 drive less than other drivers, they have more accidents per mile. According to the American Automobile Association, those over 65 are 3.5 times more likely to be killed when involved in a two-car accident. They tend to be most deficient in the following areas:

- They may be less flexible physically and sometimes fail to look behind them when changing lanes.
- Older drivers tend to travel on secondary routes, which are more dangerous than highways.
- As you age, your eyes may take longer to focus, thus making night driving especially hazardous.
- Many older drivers learned to drive before driver-education courses existed. Obtain a copy of the current driver's manual and brush up.

6 Certain food combinations interfere with your digestion.

False. Despite the popularity of "food-combining" theories, such as those restricting the combination of proteins and fats or starches in one meal, there is no evidence that any type of food should not be combined with another. Most foods, in fact, are already natural combinations of fat, protein and carbohydrate even when eaten alone. And overwhelming evidence recommends a varied, balanced diet as the most healthful. Studies show that most vitamins and minerals are best utilized when consumed as part of a complex mixture of foods.

7 Exercise cannot undo the effects of a high-cholesterol diet.

True. Regular aerobic exercise such as running, swimming or cycling can reduce your overall cholesterol level slightly, and raise the protective HDL component. Unless combined with a sensible eating plan, exercise alone will not have a significant impact on your cholesterol levels.

In a recent study, 10 men with low cholesterol levels engaged in a vigorous, 25-minute aerobic exercise program four times a week. They also maintained a diet low in saturated fat and moderately low in total fat. When the men consumed 600 milligrams of cholesterol daily, their blood cholesterol levels rose sharply. Returning to a low-cholesterol diet reduced their blood cholesterol to normal levels.

8 A vasectomy involves little or no risk.

True. While a 1978 study showed that vasectomized monkeys tended to develop atherosclerosis faster than nonvasectomized ones when both groups were fed a high-fat diet, no study has shown a similar effect on humans. One study examined the health records of 10,590 men for as long as 40 years after the procedure and found no evidence of increased risk of heart disease or any other health concern.

9 Too much close-up work can hurt a child's eyes.

False. While it is possible that an excessive amount of close-up work can disrupt eye growth and cause nearsightedness, this disorder is far more likely to be caused by genetic factors. Do not worry if your children enjoy close-up work. Make sure that they have good light and rest their eyes periodically by looking into the distance. Any child who complains of blurred vision should be examined by an ophthalmologist.

10 Drunk drivers get hurt in accidents less often than sober drivers.

False. Drunk drivers are involved in far more accidents than sober drivers and they are more likely to be injured or killed. In one study of more than a million crashes, it was determined that drunk drivers were injured or killed more often than sober ones. The injuries of the intoxicated subjects were likely to be worse and their head injuries were more often fatal, because alcohol makes brain tissue swell. The drunk drivers tended to sustain more severe injuries even in low-speed, low-damage crashes, which suggests that the mere presence of alcohol in the blood enhances the degree of any injury.

11 Diet sodas and artificial sweeteners can actually make you gain weight.

True. There is no evidence that eating artificially sweetened foods or drinking diet sodas will help you lose weight. A study by the American Cancer Society suggests, however, that those who consume sugar substitutes actually tend to gain more weight than those who do not use them. There are two reasons for this. First, artificial sweeteners do not replace high-calorie, high-fat foods; they are simply used in addition to them. Those who would not add a teaspoon of sugar to their coffee, for instance, might still eat a fruit-flavored yogurt, which may contain over six teaspoons of sugar. Second, artificial sweeteners do not suppress appetite; they actually increase hunger in many people, leading them to consume more calories than they would if they simply had a sugar food.

A better bet for losing weight is a regular exercise program and a moderately calorie-restricted diet that emphasizes complex carbohydrates such as fruits, vegetables and whole grains.

12 Fasting will not help you lose weight permanently or rid your body of toxins.

True. There is no evidence that fasting can cleanse your body or lead to permanent weight reduction. While fasting may lead to rapid initial weight loss, most of that is fluid. As the fast continues, you may lose some fat, but most of the loss will be lean tissue such as muscle. Soon your metabolism will slow down, and the rate of weight loss will decrease.

Few people who fast to lose weight are able to maintain their weight loss, since they regain it as soon as they begin eating again, and some may sustain permanent injury as a result of lost muscle and minerals. Although there is usually no danger in fasting for 24 hours as long as you are in good health, it will not yield any permanent benefits.

13 Herbal tea is safer for you than regular tea or coffee.

False. The FDA has warned that some herbal teas may contain substances that are considerably more hazardous than anything in coffee or regular tea. While the herbs in most packaged teas appear to be harmless, some of their ingredients may cause adverse reactions. Chamomile, a common ingredient, causes allergic reactions in people sensitive to ragweed and goldenrod. Sassafras, also widely found in herbal teas, is a known carcinogen. Nutmeg, another herbal tea additive, is toxic in large quantities.

Your Medical Age

This test has been developed to allow you to compare your medical age, a theoretical computation based on various risk factors, with your actual age. It is designed to stimulate your thinking about your lifestyle habits and preventive medicine. The scoring is based on statistical generalizations of health and longevity. Because no test can possibly take every health risk into account, and because some of the questions are based on self-evaluations, which may not be reliable, you should consider your medical age to be more of a guide than a precise measurement. Even so, the results offer a general idea of how your lifestyle and health habits affect your longevity. For greatest accuracy, the test should only be taken by persons over 25 who are in good health.

How To Take the Test:

Read each entry and determine your answer based on the number given in the parenthesis. Write your score on the lines provided in the plus or minus columns. If you are uncertain about an answer, leave it blank. At the end of each section, add up the plus and minus columns, then combine the two numbers to obtain a single subtotal. At the end of the test, follow the instructions for calculating your medical age.

Interpreting the Results:

It is best to score as low as possible on this test. If your medical age exceeds your current age, it is time to evaluate your lifestyle to seek improvements. Take the Health-Risk-Assessment Questionnaire in the following section, then turn to the appropriate topics in this book for useful tips on how to reduce your health risks. If your medical age is lower than your actual age, you may feel encouraged to continue making healthy lifestyle choices and perhaps lower your medical age even further. Once you have adopted the recommended measures, you may find it helpful to take this test occasionally to re-evaluate your medical age.

PERSONAL HISTORY	+	−
1 Your weight at age 20 was _____ . If your current weight is within 10 pounds of your weight at age 20, score (-3). If your current weight is between 10 and 20 pounds heavier, score (0). If your current weight is more than 20 pounds over your weight at age 20, score (+6) for every 20 pounds.	___	___
2 If you are under 40: Your blood pressure is above 130/80 mm/Hg (+12). Over 40: It is above 140/90 mm/Hg (+12).	___	___
3 If you are under 40: Your total cholesterol level is above 220 ml/dl (+6). Over 40: It is above 250 ml/dl (+6).	___	___
4 You have a heart murmur that is not an "innocent" type (+24).	___	___
5 You have a heart murmur with a history of rheumatic fever (+48).	___	___
6 You have had bacterial pneumonia more than three times (+6).	___	___
7 You have asthma (+6).	___	___
8 You have rectal polyps (+6).	___	___
9 You have adult-onset diabetes (+18).	___	___
10 You have severe, frequent periods of depression (+12).	___	___
11 You have regular,° complete medical checkups (-12); partial checkups (-6).	___	___
12 You have dental checkups twice a year (-3).	___	___
SUBTOTAL	___ − ___ =

°At least every four to five years before age 40, every four years between 40 and 50, every two years between 50 and 60, and every year after 60.

LIFESTYLE | + | −

1 You are good natured and easygoing (-3); you have an average disposition (0); you are tense and nervous most of the time (+6). _____ _____

2 You are physically active at work or you have a well-planned, vigorous aerobic exercise program (-12); you have a sedentary job but you exercise moderately and regularly (0); you do sedentary work and do not exercise (+12). _____ _____

3 Your family life is usually pleasant (-6); average (0); usually tense (+9). _____ _____

4 Your level of job satisfaction is above average (-3); average (0); below average (+6). _____ _____

5 You are regularly exposed to substantial air pollution (+9). _____ _____

6 You are a nonsmoker (-6); you smoke a pipe or cigars, or smoke a pack or less of cigarettes daily (+12); you smoke more than a pack of cigarettes daily (+24). _____ _____

7 You seldom drink alcohol (-6); you drink less than two beers or eight ounces of wine or two ounces of liquor daily (+6); you drink more than that amount (+24). _____ _____

8 You only drink skim or low-fat milk (-3); your diet is high in whole-grain foods, vegetables and starches (-3); you consume meat three times daily (+6); you use more than two pats of butter daily (+6); you drink more than four cups of coffee, tea or cola daily (+6); you usually add salt to foods at the table (+6). _____ _____

9 You regularly drive less than 20,000 miles annually and always wear a seat belt (-3); you drive less than 20,000 but only wear your seat belt sometimes (0); you drive more than 20,000 annually (+12). _____ _____

10 You use marijuana (+24); you use other drugs such as cocaine or heroin (+36). _____ _____

SUBTOTAL _____ − _____ =

FAMILY AND SOCIAL HISTORY | + | −

1 Your father is alive and over 68, for each five years above 68 (-3); your father is younger than 68, or he died after 68 (0); your father died of medical causes (not from an accident) before 68 (+3). _____ _____

2 Your mother is alive and over 73, for each five years above 73 (-3); your mother is younger than 68, or she died after 68 (0); your mother died of medical causes (not from an accident) before 73 (+3). _____ _____

3 You are married (0); you are unmarried and over 40 (+6). _____ _____

4 You live in a large city (+6); suburb (0); farm or small town (-3). _____ _____

SUBTOTAL _____ − _____ =

FOR WOMEN | + | −

1 Your mother or any of your sisters or maternal aunts has had breast cancer (+6). _____ _____

2 You examine your breasts monthly (-6). _____ _____

3 You are under 40 and have a breast exam performed by a physician every three years, or you are over 40 and have a breast exam every year (-6). _____ _____

4 You have an annual Pap smear (-6). _____ _____

SUBTOTAL _____ − _____ =

CALCULATIONS:
Step 1: Combine all of the totals in the yellow circles and arrive at a plus or minus number. For example: -6 -24 +6 -12 = -36 **Step 2:** Divide that number by +12 (remember that when you divide a minus number by a plus number, the result will be a minus number). For example: -36 ÷ +12 = -3 **Step 3:** Combine this number with your current age. For example: -3 + 43 = 40 The result is your medical age.

13

Health-Risk-Assessment Questionnaire

The following questions are designed to increase your knowledge and awareness of your overall health. They will not tell you how precisely you compare to the rest of the population, but the scoring chart at the end will show you the areas where you are making healthy choices and the ones that need improvement. Answer each question by circling the letter indicating yes or no. If you cannot answer the question, do not circle either; go on to the next question. At the end of each section, add up the number of answers in each column.

A PHYSICAL FITNESS

1 Do you perform aerobic exercise or engage in a vigorous sport for at least 30 minutes three times a week?   Y   N

2 Do you warm up before exercising and cool down afterward?   Y   N

3 Do you use — and replace when worn out — appropriate gear, safety equipment and shoes made specifically for your sport or activity?   Y   N

4 Whenever possible, do you walk or ride a bicycle instead of drive?   Y   N

5 Do you use stairs instead of escalators or elevators whenever possible?   Y   N

6 Are you in better shape and more vigorous than most other people your age?   Y   N

7 Do you enjoy outdoor activities, even in the winter?   Y   N

8 Do you sometimes enter athletic competitions such as cycling or foot races, fun runs or walkathons?   Y   N

TOTALS

B WEIGHT CONTROL

1 Are you ashamed of your appearance or weight?   N   Y

2 Do you ever take diet pills?   N   Y

3 Do you diet frequently and fail?   N   Y

4 Do you include exercise in your weight-control plan?   Y   N

5 Have you ever lost weight on a diet but gained it all back again?   N   Y

6 Do you feel that you would be happy and successful if only you were thin?   N   Y

7 Have you ever vomited deliberately or taken a laxative to avoid gaining weight?   N   Y

TOTALS

C   EATING HABITS

1	Do you add salt to foods during cooking and at the table?	N	Y
2	Do you drink two or more soft drinks a day?	N	Y
3	Do you eat fish and poultry more often than red meat?	Y	N
4	Do you eat high-fiber foods such as vegetables, fruits and whole grains several times a day?	Y	N
5	Do you eat sugary or salty snacks?	N	Y
6	Do you often eat ice cream, frosted cake, doughnuts or pie?	N	Y
7	Do you eat daily servings of cholesterol-rich foods such as eggs, liver and fatty meat?	N	Y
8	Do you eat a lot of saturated fat such as whole-milk dairy products, fried foods and fatty meat?	N	Y

TOTALS

D   SAFETY

		N	Y
1	Do you drive after drinking alcohol or using other drugs, or ride with drivers who have?	N	Y
2	Have you received a ticket for speeding or any other moving violation within the last two years?	N	Y
3	Do you use a radar detector to avoid speed traps when you drive?	N	Y
4	Do you wear your seat belt at all times?	Y	N
5	Do you periodically take your car in for routine maintenance?	Y	N
6	Do you ride a motorcycle or an all-terrain vehicle?	N	Y
7	Do you wear a helmet when riding a bike or motorcycle?	Y	N
8	Do you smoke in bed?	N	Y
9	Have you conducted a radon test in your home?	Y	N
10	Do the members of your family know what to do in case someone chokes on his food or stops breathing?	Y	N
11	Do you keep a gun in the house?	N	Y
12	Are you informed and careful when using potentially harmful products or substances such as household cleaners, poisons, flammables, solvents, power tools and other electrical devices?	Y	N
13	During the past year, were you involved in or a witness to two or more fights or attacks?	N	Y

TOTALS

E HEART HEALTH

1 Do you smoke cigarettes?   N   Y

2 Do you know what your cholesterol level is?   Y   N

3 If you do know your total cholesterol level, is it below 200 mg/dl?   Y   N

4 Is your average blood pressure over 140/84 mm/Hg?   N   Y

5 Is there heart disease in your family?   N   Y

6 Do any of your relatives take medication for hypertension or high cholesterol?   N   Y

7 Do you exercise regularly?   Y   N

8 Are you overweight?   N   Y

9 Do you ever feel chest pain, nausea or dizziness when you perform sudden or
  unusual exertion such as running for a bus or shoveling snow?   N   Y

10 Do you have diabetes?   N   Y

                                                                              TOTALS

F PREVENTING CANCER

1 Is there a history of cancer in your family?   N   Y

2 Do you smoke?   N   Y

3 Do you avoid getting sunburned or a dark tan?   Y   N

4 Do you have a physician look at moles or spots on your skin that are growing
  or changing?   Y   N

5 Do you have a history of sexually transmitted disease?   N   Y

6 Do fatty foods take up a large percentage of your regular diet?   N   Y

7 Are you overweight?   N   Y

8 Do you exercise at least three times a week?   Y   N

9 Do you eat high-fiber foods such as whole grains and vegetables?   Y   N

                                                                              TOTALS

G SELF-CARE

1 Do you brush and floss your teeth daily?   Y   N

2 Do you have a dental checkup at least once a year?   Y   N

3 Do you usually get an adequate amount of sleep?   Y   N

4 Do you use sunscreen and avoid excessive exposure to the sun?   Y   N

5 Do you have a personal physician?   Y   N

6 Do you avoid having unnecessary X-rays?   Y   N

7 Have you had your blood pressure checked in the past year?   Y   N

8 Do you suffer from chronic pain such as headache or backache?   N   Y

9 For women: Have you had a Pap smear within the last two years?   Y   N

10 For women: Do you examine your breasts for unusual changes or lumps at least
once a month?   Y   N

11 For men: Do you examine your testicles for unusual changes or lumps at least
once every three months?   Y   N

12 If you are over 40: Have you had a test for glaucoma within the last four years?   Y   N

13 If you are over 40: Have you had a test for hidden blood in your stool within the
last two years? If you are over 50: Have you been tested within the last year?   Y   N

14 If you are over 50: Have you had at least one sigmoidoscopy of the lower bowel?   Y   N

                                                                                        TOTALS

H INFECTIOUS DISEASES

1 Do you suffer from frequent colds and infections?   N   Y

2 Are you casual about personal hygiene?   N   Y

3 Do you have young children?   N   Y

4 Do you wash your hands frequently when you have a cold, or when people you live
or work with have colds?   Y   N

5 Has your tap water ever been checked for bacterial contamination?   Y   N

6 Do you have multiple sexual partners?   N   Y

7 Is your nutrition adequate?   Y   N

8 Are you immunized against diphtheria, measles, mumps, rubella and tetanus?   Y   N

9 Do you take antibiotics whenever you catch a cold or the flu?   N   Y

                                                                                        TOTALS

I EMOTIONAL HEALTH

1	Are you able to fall asleep when you want to and wake up refreshed in the morning?	Y	N
2	During the past year, have you suffered a personal loss or misfortune such as the death of someone close to you, the loss of your job, divorce or disability?	N	Y
3	Are you generally satisfied with your life?	Y	N
4	Do you include time to relax as part of your daily routine?	Y	N
5	Do you make time for friends and family?	Y	N
6	Are you satisfied with your level of sexual activity?	Y	N
7	Are you satisfied with your sexual relationships?	Y	N

TOTALS

J CIGARETTES, ALCOHOL AND OTHER DRUGS

1	Do you smoke cigarettes, cigars or pipes, or do you chew tobacco?	N	Y
2	Do you ever take recreational drugs such as marijuana or cocaine?	N	Y
3	Do you drink alcohol frequently?	N	Y
4	If you drink, do you limit yourself to two drinks a day?	Y	N
5	Do you ever try to hide your alcohol or drug use?	N	Y
6	Have you ever tried to stop drinking, smoking or taking drugs and failed?	N	Y
7	Have family members, coworkers or friends ever commented about your drinking or using drugs?	N	Y
8	Have you ever missed work or called in sick because of drinking or drugs?	N	Y
9	Do you feel you need to drink or to take a drug before you go to a party or meet other people socially?	N	Y
10	Do you find you need to confine your drinking or drug taking to specific times of the day or days of the week in order to control it?	N	Y
11	Do you ever ignore the label directions when using prescription and over-the-counter drugs?	N	Y

TOTALS

Scoring

For each section, write the number of answers you marked in the lefthand column in the blanks below.

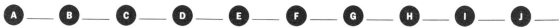

A — B — C — D — E — F — G — H — I — J —

Section G: Add one point to your total if you are female; add two if you are male. In addition, add three points if you are under 40; add two if you are under 50.

Section J: Add one point if you do not drink alcohol at all.

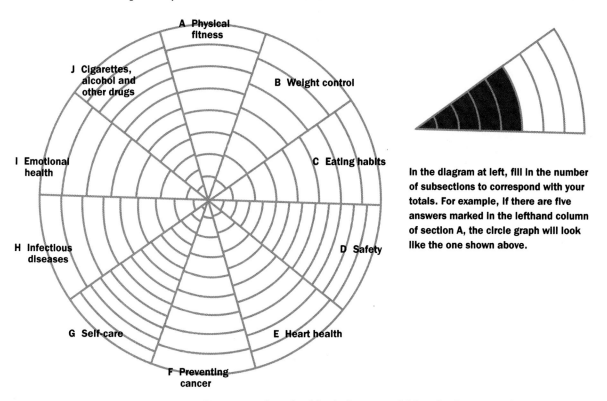

In the diagram at left, fill in the number of subsections to correspond with your totals. For example, if there are five answers marked in the lefthand column of section A, the circle graph will look like the one shown above.

Sections that are completely shaded: You are making healthy behavior and lifestyle choices in these areas. Keep up the good work and use this book as an occasional reference.

Sections that are partially shaded: Look up the appropriate topics in this book for tips on improving your health-risk profiles in these areas. With a little more awareness and effort, you could not only live a healthier life, but a longer one, too.

Sections that are barely shaded or not shaded at all: There is significant room for increasing your health and satisfaction in these areas. Use this book to help you work first on those areas where you are most likely to be successful, then tackle the tougher sections.

Note: For a variety of reasons, you may never be able to shade in certain sections completely. For instance, you do not have control over your family history. Sections that you may never be able to shade in should alert you to be more diligent in the other areas in which you do have more control.

The Step Test

The questionnaire on the preceding pages indicates your health and lifestyle habits. This three-minute step test evaluates your aerobic fitness. All you need is a stopwatch or wristwatch with a second hand and an eight-inch-high step or stool. The results indicate your heart's ability to recover from mild exertion. A quick recovery is considered by physiologists to be a sign of fitness.

Although it is not meant to diagnose heart problems, the test is a useful tool for determining your present level of fitness. Taken once a month, it can also be a measure of your improvement in an aerobic exercise program. The test is quite safe for healthy individuals. However, people who have any heart trouble or those over 35 who have not exercised regularly for a year or more should consult a physician before performing the test.

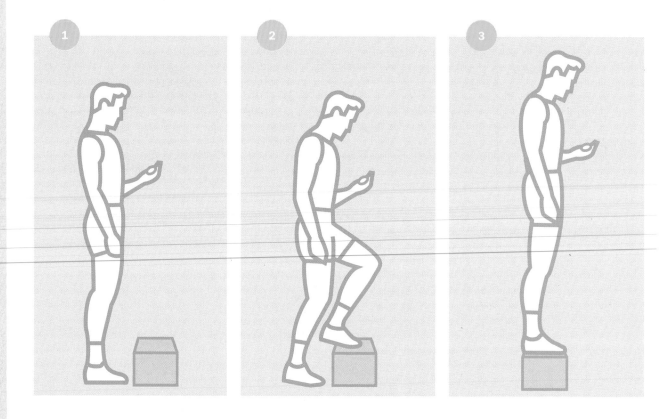

Stand in front of an eight-inch-high step or stool and step up and down in the sequence shown above. Perform two cycles every five seconds for three minutes, then sit down and rest for 30 seconds. Find your pulse in the radial artery in your wrist, then count it for 30 seconds. Compare the result with the chart at right.

Step Test Results

MEN				
Age 20-29	30-39	40-49	50 & older	**Your classification**
NUMBER OF HEARTBEATS				
34-36	35-38	37-39	37-40	Excellent
37-40	39-41	40-42	41-43	Good
41-42	42-43	43-44	44-45	Average
43-47	44-47	45-49	46-49	Fair
48-59	48-59	50-60	50-62	Poor

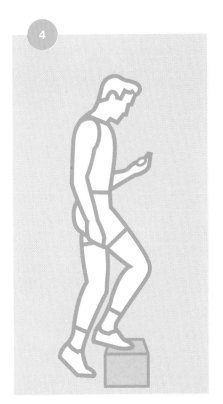

WOMEN				
Age 20-29	30-39	40-49	50 & older	**Your classification**
NUMBER OF HEARTBEATS				
38-42	39-42	41-43	41-44	Excellent
43-44	43-45	44-45	45-47	Good
45-46	46-47	46-47	48-49	Average
47-52	48-53	48-54	50-55	Fair
53-66	54-66	55-67	56-66	Poor

If the result of your step test is poor or fair, you definitely need to begin an aerobic exercise program; be sure to follow the directions on pages 84-85. If your result is average, you should exercise more regularly; perform at least a 20-minute routine three times a week. If your result is good, you are in good shape, but there is still room for improvement; increase the intensity or duration of your workouts. If your result is excellent, continue with your fitness regimen.

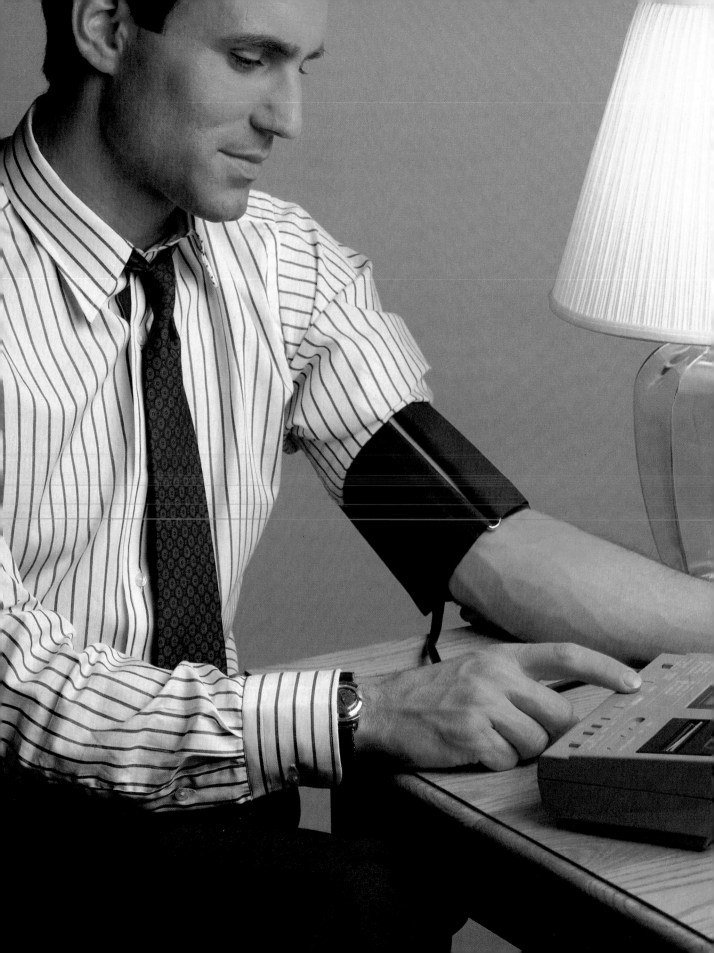

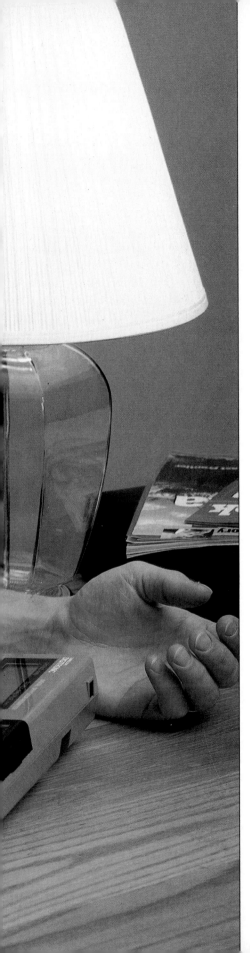

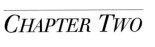

CHAPTER TWO

Longevity

Understanding health risks

T he first and foremost goal of wellness is preventing illness, especially those health problems that can shorten your life. This chapter covers the nine leading causes of mortality in the United States today — including the latest medical information, the predisposing risk factors and the steps that you can take to reduce your risks.

Through the years, the conditions that affect longevity have changed significantly. At the turn of the century in the United States, influenza, pneumonia, diphtheria, tuberculosis and gastrointestinal infections were the major illnesses that caused the most fatalities. Although the development of penicillin and vaccinations did much to reduce the incidence of most of these illnesses, the mortality rate from such diseases as typhoid, pneumonia and diphtheria had already plunged dramatically by the time many of the most effective medical therapies had been developed. Improved medicines have been re-sponsible for only a 10-percent reduction in the rate of infectious

23

diseases and 3.5-percent decline in deaths from communicable diseases since 1900.

Actually, these diseases were eliminated by other changes and improvements that, for the most part, are now taken for granted. Dramatic reductions in the mortality rate from infectious diseases from 1900 to 1920 were realized largely by improvements in nutrition and sanitation through the widespread introduction of electricity, refrigeration, running water, sewage disposal and many other conveniences. Refrigeration not only helped prevent contamination of food by bacteria and fungi, it allowed long-term storage and cross-country transportation of food products, thereby helping to prevent nutritional deficiencies. Largely because of this public-health revolution, life expectancy increased from 49 in 1900 to 70 in 1966. By the time antibiotics and vaccines were developed — mostly after 1940 — life expectancy had already increased significantly and had begun to level off.

Today in Western societies, communicable diseases are generally not a source of significant mortality. Although people may fear an infectious disease such as AIDS, they are much more likely to suffer a heart attack, stroke, cancer or emphysema — the current leading causes of death. Medical researchers still do not completely understand the biochemistry of these problems — for example, what causes a cell to be cancerous or plaque to accumulate in arteries — but they have determined some of the principle risk factors that promote the illnesses. And, as was true of communicable diseases, changing patterns of behavior and lifestyle play crucial roles. The difference is that, whereas the previously most feared diseases were aggravated by deficiencies — in food, vitamins and sanitation — many of today's fatal conditions are caused or exacerbated by excesses. Numerous studies in recent years have shown a correlation between heart disease, cancer, hypertension, stroke and other health problems and excessive consumption of calories, fat, cholesterol, alcohol and the practice of unhealthy habits such as smoking. Likewise, while physical hardship hampered the health of people at the turn of the century, today the problem is a sedentary lifestyle.

As these risk factors have become publicized, some of them have already been reduced, which suggests that Americans may indeed be incorporating the principles of wellness into their lives. According to a report from the National Centers for Disease Control, the mortality rate for heart disease and stroke fell 18 percent and 26 percent, respectively, between 1979 and 1986. Although better medical care certainly contributed to this improvement, research has indicated that lifestyle changes had the most significant impact. During that period, for example, increasing numbers of adult Americans reduced their intake of such fatty foods as eggs, beef and butter; they smoked fewer cigarettes; and they began exercising regularly.

There is still much that Americans can do to improve their health. While most people say they are concerned about cholesterol, for instance, 90 percent of Americans do not know what their cholesterol levels are or how much of this artery-clogging substance is collecting in their veins. And despite the well-documented benefits of exercise, 80 percent of Americans are either completely sedentary or exercise so infrequently that it produces few results. While many people do not consume as much red meat, whole milk and other high-fat products, fat continues to supply 42 percent of the calories in the average American diet, which is more than that found in almost any other society. In addition, cholesterol levels remain far too high among an estimated 60 million people in the United States.

Americans also suffer from an extraordinarily high rate of chemical addictions — many more than from the heroin, cocaine, angel dust and other exotic and sometimes lethal substances that are available on the streets of virtually every city. Actually, legal substances — tobacco, alcohol and a host of prescription drugs — cause the most destructive addictions. Although more people than ever before have given up cigarettes, millions more still smoke. Despite extensive and costly national health-education campaigns, smoking remains the number-one cause of preventable death in America.

In addition to diet, exercise and avoiding toxic substances, safety precautions have also become an increasingly important aspect of wellness. While technology has improved our health, many individuals subject themselves to numerous risks of physical injuries. Many people ski down steep slopes, drive automobiles at high speeds without air bags or seat belts, use power tools, store toxic chemicals in their houses and have access to guns. Nearly 100,000 people die annually from accidents. While it is neither possible nor likely that people will eliminate all of these high-technology health risks, it is entirely possible to reduce the chance of injury and death by training adequately, taking appropriate precautions and always using the safest equipment. For instance, if people made a habit of using seat belts in cars, thousands of lives could be saved annually.

If you have taken the Health-Risk-Assessment Questionnaire on pages 14 to 19, you presumably know which areas of your lifestyle habits need to be improved. The topics in this chapter will help you identify your most important concerns. For instance, if you know you have high blood pressure, or if anyone in your family has been diagnosed as having hypertension, the chart on page 35 is relevant to you. It indicates that regular exercise and a balanced diet will help you lower your blood pressure.

Each chart also refers you to related topics for practical information on improving your health profile. For instance, if stress is contributing to your high blood pressure, the chart refers you to a section on stress management. Similarly, each of the nine health-risk sections identifies many of the factors that contribute to preventable risks, or suggests lifestyle factors that may protect you from them; in each case, you are referred to appropriate topics that provide tips for improving wellness.

Addictions

No one ever chooses to become addicted to anything; nevertheless, barely a single family is untouched by someone with an addiction. Indeed, addiction is so pervasive in every social and economic class that one medical historian calls it "the American disease."

Addictions include chemical dependencies on a wide variety of substances, which are characterized by increased tolerance for the drug so that the user must ingest ever-increasing doses to achieve the same effect. Depending on the substance, withdrawal may induce feelings of anxiety, restlessness, irritability and drug craving. Narcotic withdrawal can result in severe symptoms that include convulsions and even cardiovascular collapse.

In recent years, though, addictions have come to mean psychological dependence as well as purely physical dependence on a chemical. Some researchers believe that many of the same mechanisms that govern chemical addictions also seem to operate for compulsive and self-destructive behavioral addictions, which include compulsive overeating, gambling, sex and shopping.

The most commonly abused addictive drugs are not heroin or cocaine but cigarettes and alcohol. One study indicates that nicotine, which is inhaled along with 4,000 other chemicals and gases, is the most powerfully addictive drug of all. Tobacco is also the most destructive drug, possibly causing as many as 400,000 deaths a year in the United States and costing approximately $65 billion in health-care bills and lost productivity.

Nearly half of the American public drinks alcohol; and 10 percent of the population is addicted to it. Alcoholics account for 20 percent of all hospital admissions. The health-care costs and lost productivity amount to $15 billion a year.

Many people overuse caffeine, a mild stimulant that is found in coffee, tea, cola, chocolate and many nonprescription drugs. Caffeine can cause an irregular heartbeat and elevated blood pressure.

Although thousands of people die annually from their addictions, most deaths are never attributed to their habits. The fatalities are often considered to be suicides, accidents, heart failures, cirrhosis of the liver or a variety of other ailments. There is no measurement for the terrible emotional anguish suffered by addicts and their families.

Because many addicts try to give up their habits and fail, they often feel that trying to quit is hopeless. However, between 1964 and 1985, 32 million Americans managed to shake one of the toughest addictions of all — nicotine. No matter what the addiction, only about 20 percent of those who try to kick a habit succeed on the first attempt.

If your problem is alcohol, then you can turn to your local chapter of Alcoholics Anonymous. If you are a smoker, call the American Cancer Society or the American Lung Association for a stop-smoking clinic. Joining a self-help group and substituting a positive addiction such as regular exercise are often the strongest predictors of kicking a chemical or psychological dependency. The chart (right) explains the effects of four of the most commonly abused substances; it also refers you to pages that can help you overcome these habits.

Effects of Commonly Abused Substances

ALCOHOL

CAFFEINE

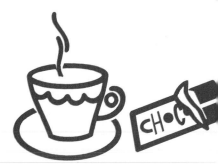

TRANQUILIZERS

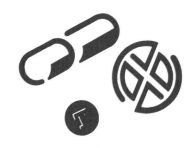

TOBACCO

AFFECTED BODY SYSTEMS

Heart, blood vessels	Brain, nervous system	Lungs, liver	Reproductive system
Reduces heart's ability to pump blood. Can damage cells of the heart muscle. Increases incidence and severity of hypertension.	Alcohol is a depressant. Slows down activity and impairs efficiency of the central nervous system, affecting behavior, mood, judgment and motor coordination. Dulls memory, learning and reasoning ability, concentration, perception and reflexes. Causes unsteady gait and reduces manual skill. High concentrations in bloodstream can cause confusion, incoordination and disorientation. May lead to stupor, anesthesia, coma or death.	Alcohol consumption is associated with a higher incidence of upper respiratory infections. Also, prolonged, heavy drinking can result in potentially fatal cirrhosis (a degeneration of the liver) and liver cancer. Drinking bouts can cause alcoholic hepatitis (an inflammation of the liver). Damages liver and interferes with its ability to absorb and store certain B vitamins.	Drinking during pregnancy can produce a set of birth defects known as fetal alcohol syndrome. Decreases levels of testosterone, impairing potency. Prolonged, excessive consumption can result in chronically low testosterone levels, causing shrinkage of the testicles and breast growth in men. To learn more about alcoholism, and for tips on how to cut down on your alcohol intake, see pages 52-53.
Can cause irregular heartbeats, or arrhythmias. Research directly linking caffeine and heart disease has proved inconclusive.	Stimulates the central nervous system, producing nervousness, trembling, irritability, throbbing headaches, disorientation, depression and insomnia in some people, often referred to as coffee nerves. More than two to four cups of coffee daily can lead to symptoms of anxiety and produce an inability to concentrate.		Studies have indicated that caffeine consumed during pregnancy can increase the risk of stillbirth and miscarriage.
Some tranquilizers can cause heart palpitations.	Slows nervous system function. Can impair reaction time, mental alertness, judgment and coordination. When taken for more than three days, they can cause lethargy during waking periods and aggravate insomnia. Protracted use can lead to fatigue and depression.	Tranquilizers can worsen severe breathing problems. Extended use of certain tranquilizers (such as diazepam, or Valium) can impair liver function. The liver converts some tranquilizers into long-acting forms (active metabolites) that can linger in the body for 24 hours or longer. When these tranquilizers are used on a daily basis for an extended period, an increased sedation may result.	Studies reveal a possible link between birth defects and use of certain tranquilizers during pregnancy.
The relationship between smoking and heart disease is firmly established. Smoking decreases levels of beneficial HDL cholesterol, speeds up heart rate and raises blood pressure.	The nicotine in tobacco may facilitate feelings of relaxation or mental acuity in nicotine-dependent individuals. However, smoking interferes with oxygen delivery to the brain. Affects a major neurotransmitter system that is involved in the conduction of nerve cells. A major cause of stroke.	Smoking is responsible for more than three-fourths of all lung cancer cases, the leading fatal cancer in the United States. Impairs functions of the respiratory system. Smokers have more difficulty keeping lungs clear of infectious organisms and harmful debris. Smokers are usually more short-winded than nonsmokers. Cigarettes account for three-fourths of the cases of chronic bronchitis and emphysema.	Smoking during pregnancy reduces the blood and oxygen supply to the fetus and increases the risk of miscarriage, premature birth, stillbirth, low birth weight and death shortly after birth. For tips on how to quit smoking, see pages 118-119.

27

Cancer

Cancer is one of the most feared diseases in America. Affecting virtually every family at some time, it is the second-leading cause of death, claiming over 450,000 victims each year. While it is more common as you age, cancer strikes randomly, afflicting people of all ages, races and socioeconomic levels. Indeed, approximately one-third of all Americans are expected to contract some sort of cancer during their lives; more than 900,000 individuals are faced with this life-threatening diagnosis annually.

Cancer need not be deadly, however; in fact, with current therapies, it is cured almost as often as not. Much of this improvement in cure rates is due to advances in cancer treatments, which, over the past two decades, have been occurring with increasing success. The usual modes of treatment are surgery, radiation therapy and chemotherapy.

Cancer is actually a general term for more than 100 different diseases characterized by the uncontrolled growth of abnormal cells. Eventually, this growth, called a neoplasm or tumor, interferes with essential bodily functions. Cancer can occur in any of the tissues or organs of the body, and it can spread by invading nearby tissues, or by traveling through the circulatory system to other parts of the body in a process called metastasis.

Early detection remains one of the best defenses against many forms of cancer; indeed, experts estimate that more than one-third of the 462,000 Americans who died of it in 1985 could have been saved by earlier diagnosis and treatment. For example, the American Cancer Society estimates that three-quarters of colon-rectal cancer — the second and third most common cancers in men and women, respectively — is curable if it is treated in the early stages.

Certain factors can increase your likelihood of contracting specific cancers. By being aware of them, you can usually reduce your risk. (*See the chart opposite.*) High-risk individuals should be monitored by their physicians, who can utilize a variety of diagnostic techniques to catch most cancers at early and treatable stages. For example, women with a history of breast cancer in their immediate families are two to three times more likely to contract it, so they should undergo more frequent diagnostic tests. With early detection and prompt treatment, about 85 percent of breast-cancer patients can be cured completely.

Take precaution by regularly examining your skin, breasts, testicles and bowel function. In addition, preventive measures in your diet and lifestyle can provide protection against the disease. The most important step is to stop smoking: 30 percent of all cancer cases and 83 percent of the incidence of lung cancer can be directly attributed to the hazards of smoking.

The connection between diet and cancer provides the most promising research to date. Studies by the National Cancer Institute estimate that one-third of all cancer cases are in some way linked to diet. You should limit fat, alcohol, nitrites (preservatives in smoked and processed meats), aflatoxins (poisons in moldy nuts, seeds and grains) and meats that are grilled, barbecued or fried. Instead, your diet should be rich in vitamins A, C and E, fiber and cruciferous vegetables such as cabbages, broccoli and cauliflower. See the chart (*right*) for links between cancer and foods or other risk factors that may lead to the disease.

The Relationship Between Cancer and Aging

Number of cases
per 100,000 people
(both sexes)

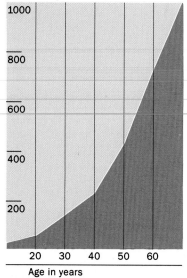

Age in years

Because the majority of cancer cases develop over many years, the disease most frequently affects people in midlife or older. As the graph above shows, the number of cases rises steadily with age. By age 70, there are 1,000 cancer cases per 100,000 men and women.

Common Forms of Cancer

	RISK FACTORS	PREVENTIVE ACTIONS
Breast	Having close relatives with breast cancer. Risk is especially great for women whose sisters or mothers had breast cancer before menopause. Early menarche and late natural menopause (the longer ovaries produce sex hormones, the greater the risk). Having a first baby after age 30 or never having one. Previous breast cancer. High-fat diets.	Many women have detected breast cancer at a curable stage by giving themselves monthly self-examinations two or three days after the end of their menstrual periods. Women should also have breast examinations at least annually by a doctor or nurse. Women who have cystic breast disease, a benign breast disorder, should have more frequent exams. To learn how to do a breast self-examination, see page 135.
Cervical	First intercourse before age 18. Multiple sex partners. Genital herpes or venereal warts. History of gonorrhea or syphilis. Five or more completed pregnancies.	Cancer of the cervix develops slowly and can easily be detected by a Pap smear and cured. The American College of Obstetricians and Gynecologists recommends that when a woman reaches 18 or becomes sexually active, she should have Pap smears for three consecutive years. Thereafter, she should be tested at the discretion of her physician. Women at risk for cervical cancer should have the test annually. To learn how to protect against sexually transmitted diseases, see pages 112-113.
Colon/Rectal	Personal or family history of colon polyps. Family history of colon or rectal cancer. Previous large-bowel cancer. History of ulcerative colitis. Low-fiber diet.	These cancers grow slowly, remaining localized for long periods and are curable for quite some time. Report rectal bleeding or any persistent changes in bowel movements to your doctor. The American Cancer Society recommends that persons over 40 should have a digital rectal examination annually. Cancer of the colon is uncommon in people whose diet is high in fresh fruits and vegetables and fish and low in saturated fat. For tips on how to increase fiber intake, see pages 82-83.
Laryngeal	Smoking. Excessive alcohol consumption. History of cancer of the lung or oral cavity.	Cancer of the larynx can be curable at an early stage. Do not smoke, and cut down on drinking alcohol. If you do smoke, refrain from drinking alcohol when smoking. For tips on how to stop smoking, see pages 118-119. To cut down on your alcohol consumption, see pages 52-53.
Lung	Cigarette smoking: the risk of developing lung cancer depends on the number of years, the quantity of cigarettes and how deeply the smoker inhales. Exposure over a long period to asbestos, chromium compounds, nickel, radioactive material or arsenic. Recurrent bouts of pneumonia. History of tuberculosis.	The best way to reduce the risk of lung cancer is to stop smoking. Even heavy smokers can lower their risk by giving up cigarettes. Avoid exposure to the cancer-causing agents listed at left. For tips on how to quit smoking, see pages 118-119.
Ovarian	Family history of ovarian cancer	Ovarian cancer rarely produces any symptoms until it has reached an advanced stage. Most women are unaware of the presence of ovarian tumors. Ovaries are checked during pelvic examinations. To find out how frequently you need to have your ovaries examined, see pages 102-103.
Prostate	Being over 50. History of two or more prostate infections. History of venereal disease.	Most men with prostate cancer have no symptoms at all. However, men over 50 should become familiar with the symptoms. The American Cancer Society recommends a digital rectal examination annually for all men over 40. This exam is the most effective test for the disease, although it does not ensure early detection.
Skin	Extremely fair complexion. Long exposure to sunlight (more than four hours a day for four months per year). Frequent or severe exposure to arsenic compounds, coal tar, radium and X-rays. Scars caused by severe burns. History of malignant moles or skin cancer. Moles on areas of the body prone to irritation by tight clothing or shaving. Moles on the soles of the feet. Scaling sores that do not heal.	Avoid sunbathing, expecially if you have a fair complexion; always use sunscreen (not regular suntan lotion or oil) and reapply it frequently. Wear protective clothing such as a hat. Avoid contact with coal tars, arsenic compounds, radium, paraffin oil and frequent exposure to X-rays. See a physician for a nonhealing sore, or for a change in the nature or size of a wart or mole. For more information on skin care, see pages 124-125.
Testicular	Undescended testicles. Exposure in the uterus to the hormone DES (used between 1940-1960 by women at risk for miscarriage). Inflammation of the testes due to mumps.	Any male born with an undescended testicle should have the condition corrected before age six. Testicular cancer is the most common malignancy in men between 25-44. Starting at 15, for early detection, men should perform testicular self-examinations once a month after a hot shower or bath. To find out how to do a testicular self-examination, see page 135.

Coronary Artery Disease

Heart disease is the number-one cause of death in the United States; among American males, it is responsible for 36 percent of all deaths. In fact, more Americans die from heart disease every year than from all forms of cancer combined.

Heart disease can strike any one of the heart's three basic systems — the valves and chambers, the heart muscle and the blood vessels that feed the muscles. The most common form of heart disease, however, is damage to the blood vessels, or coronary artery disease, which results in an impairment of the ability of the blood vessels to deliver adequate oxygen to the heart muscle.

Atherosclerosis is the most common form of coronary artery disease; it begins insidiously, perhaps as a small lesion inside a coronary artery. This lesion can be caused by damage from a virus or bacteria, or as a result of such risk factors as smoking or high cholesterol levels. This connection is not clearly understood.

Warning Signs of Coronary Artery Disease

- Chest pain that often occurs during physical exertion or bouts of emotional stress
- Shortness of breath, cold sweat, nausea
- Awakening from sleep with a sensation of choking or suffocation
- Swelling of the extremities, especially the ankles
- Erratic pulse, heart palpitations
- Fainting spells, dizziness
- Extreme fatigue with no apparent cause

According to one theory, cholesterol in the bloodstream collects on the walls of coronary arteries that feed the heart muscle and becomes trapped, where it oxidizes, turns rancid and attracts immune-system cells. Some of these scavenger cells gorge on the cholesterol, causing bulging lesions called fatty streaks.

Secretions from the cells damage the arterial walls and promote the growth of additional cells that form a scab over the lesion, which is called plaque. As more cholesterol continues to be deposited, the plaque grows and begins to impede the flow of oxygen-rich blood to the heart muscle. Eventually, it may starve portions of the heart muscle. Atherosclerosis is commonly called hardening of the arteries, and it also causes strokes and claudication, or circulation problems.

Atherosclerotic plaque can begin building up in childhood, taking many years to impair heart function. In fact, plaque often constricts 70 percent of the artery before symptoms are finally noticed. Occasionally, atherosclerosis builds without symptoms until a heart attack strikes, when a portion of the heart muscle ceases to function.

Angina pectoris, or chest pain, is a symptom of heart disease. It often occurs during times of stress or physical exertion. Typically, angina begins as a sudden pain under the breastbone that sometimes spreads to the shoulders, left arm, neck or jaw. Angina can be mild enough to be mistaken for indigestion, or it can be an intense sensation of constriction, burning or heaviness.

Atherosclerosis does not inevitably lead to a heart attack or a life debilitated by angina. Many factors affect the process: Some are givens, such as age, sex and family history. However, studies show that you can dramatically reduce your risk of coronary artery disease and heart attack by avoiding, controlling or correcting other risk factors. (See the chart opposite.) It may even be possible to reverse the disease by making certain lifestyle changes. In fact, the U.S. Public Health Service reports that the death rates from coronary artery disease declined 31 percent between 1970 and 1986. This is believed to be largely the result of stopping smoking, improving dietary habits and controlling hypertension.

Researchers believe that death from coronary artery disease can be reduced further by additional lifestyle changes. One of the most promising avenues is for people with high blood cholesterol levels to reduce them. The Lipid Research Clinic's Coronary Primary Prevention Trial determined that participants in the study who reduced their cholesterol levels by only 9 percent were able to cut their risk of heart disease by almost 20 percent.

Lowering cholesterol can often be accomplished through a sensible diet that emphasizes whole grains, fresh fruits and vegetables, without fried foods, fatty meats and products high in saturated fats and cholesterol. Have your cholesterol level and your blood pressure checked periodically by a doctor to ensure that you are maintaining a low-risk profile.

Two important lifestyle changes you can make to reduce your risk of coronary artery disease are to perform vigorous exercise regularly and control your weight. See the page references in the chart (opposite) to reduce or eliminate your risk factors.

Controllable Factors of Coronary Artery Disease

CIGARETTE SMOKING

The link between smoking and heart disease is well established. Even smoking one to four cigarettes daily can double your risk of heart attack or fatal coronary artery disease. A smoker is two to four times more likely to die from sudden cardiac arrest than a nonsmoker. Smokers are also most likely to lead sedentary lifestyles. Quitting cigarette smoking can greatly reduce the risk of coronary artery disease. For tips on how to quit, see pages 118-119.

HIGH BLOOD PRESSURE

Also called hypertension, this disease is a major factor in coronary artery disease and heart attack. Blood pressure can be controlled with diet and exercise: Being overweight increases the risk of developing high blood pressure; regular exercise is linked with lowering blood pressure. Also, excessive alcohol consumption may lead to hypertension. For tips on how to control your weight, see pages 130-131. See aerobic exercise on pages 84-85. While lifestyle changes can often reduce moderate or borderline hypertension, medications are often necessary to control severe high blood pressure.

HIGH BLOOD CHOLESTEROL

A high concentration of cholesterol in the blood often results in the formation of arterial plaque, a buildup of fatty deposits that can restrict blood flow and starve portions of the heart muscle. Cholesterol levels can be lowered by limiting the intake of dietary cholesterol and saturated fat. The consumption of soluble fiber, found in oat bran and many fresh fruits and vegetables, may also help to lower cholesterol levels. Regular aerobic exercise is beneficial in preventing obesity, which is associated with high cholesterol levels. Regular aerobic exercise also increases the blood level of protective HDL cholesterol. HDL levels can also be elevated by quitting smoking. For tips on how to control cholesterol, see pages 64-65. To cut down on saturated fat intake, see pages 80-81. To quit smoking, see pages 118-119. Tips on increasing your fiber intake are on pages 82-83.

DIABETES

Blood vessels may be damaged by diabetes, making them susceptible to the buildup of fatty deposits, called plaque, and subsequent narrowing. Type-II diabetes, the adult-onset form of the disease, which accounts for 90 percent of all diabetics, is linked with the development of heart disease. Diabetics often have high blood pressure, another risk factor for coronary artery disease. Refer to pages 32-33 for information on the control and treatment of diabetes.

OBESITY

Generally, the more overweight you are, the higher your blood pressure and serum cholesterol and triglyceride levels. Obesity is often the result of a sedentary lifestyle, which is another controllable risk factor. Weight control may avert the onset of type-II diabetes in susceptible individuals. For tips on how to control your weight, see pages 130-131.

LACK OF EXERCISE

A sedentary lifestyle is often associated with coronary artery disease. Those who do not exercise are more likely to have other risk factors associated with heart disease. Evidence shows that regular aerobic exercise helps to prevent coronary artery disease by maintaining ideal body weight and lowering blood pressure and cholesterol levels. Exercise may also encourage the formation of additional capillaries to the heart muscle, although this has not yet been proven. See aerobic exercise on pages 84-85.

STRESS

Although not a direct cause of heart disease, stress has been shown to increase hypertension and blood cholesterol levels. Studies show that persons with type-A personalities — characterized by an inability to deal with stressful situations — have a higher-than-average incidence of heart attack. According to the National Heart, Lung and Blood Institute, reducing stress helps to protect against heart disease. For tips on how to relax, see pages 122-123.

Diabetes

Warning Signs of Diabetes

TYPE I

- **Excessive thirst and urination**
- **Rapid weight loss**
- **Abnormal hunger**
- **Nausea and vomiting**
- **Fatigue, weakness, irritability**

TYPE II

- **Any of the type-I symptoms**
- **Tingling sensations, numbness or pain in the hands, feet or legs**
- **Frequent infections of the skin, urinary tract and gums**
- **Slow healing of bruises and cuts**
- **Persistent itching, especially in the genital area**
- **Blurred vision**

Diabetes is a serious and potentially life-threatening disease affecting more than 11 million Americans — almost half of whom are not even aware of having it. And the incidence of diabetes is on a rapid rise: Experts estimate that the number of diagnosed cases will double in the next decade. While it can be controlled, diabetes is incurable; indeed, because of its complications, it is the seventh-leading cause of death in America.

Diabetes results most often from your body's inability to produce insulin or to use it properly, which is essential to the conversion of food into the energy that powers virtually every cell in your body. Normally, the simple and complex carbohydrates that you eat are changed into glucose, which is carried through the bloodstream to your cells, where insulin metabolism enables your cells to convert the glucose into energy or to store it.

The lack of insulin results in a buildup of glucose in your blood. Check the warning signs in the box *(left)* for the symptoms. Ignoring them not only strains your kidneys, it can result in dehydration and excessive blood sugar that might lead to a coma.

The malabsorption of glucose can have other equally serious consequences: Without glucose, your body uses fat cells for an alternative source of energy. However, in metabolizing fat, your liver releases ketones, which can accumulate in your blood, resulting in diabetic acidosis, another potentially fatal condition.

Finally, premature hardening of the arteries and a thickening of the small blood vessels can result in blindness, heart and kidney disease, stroke, nerve damage and circulatory problems. These complications are more likely to plague diabetics later in their lives. Tragically, four out of five diabetics eventually die from cardiovascular complications.

Diabetes has two main forms: type I, insulin dependent, also known as juvenile-onset diabetes, and type II, non-insulin dependent, or adult-onset diabetes. Approximately one million people are afflicted with type-I diabetes, which usually strikes during childhood or adolescence. The pancreas either stops making insulin or makes only a tiny amount. It requires a balanced meal plan and lifelong daily insulin injections.

Type-II diabetes affects more people, but is more easily controlled. Usually a prescribed diet and exercise regimen is sufficient, although oral medication or insulin injections may be required in some cases. Weight loss is often necessary to bring the disease under control.

While your family history, age and sex affect your likelihood of contracting type-II diabetes, obesity is one of the most predisposing factors. More than 80 percent of adult diabetics are overweight. What you eat may also have some bearing on your risk of contracting it. In studies, diets high in sugar have repeatedly been linked to the onset of diabetes.

Diets high in fiber and complex carbohydrates may help reduce blood-sugar levels. Maintaining a well-balanced, healthful diet and watching your weight will delay or prevent the onset of diabetes. Regular exercise helps diabetics in two ways: It aids in weight loss and lowers blood-sugar levels. Indeed, insulin requirements seem to decrease in diabetics who exercise.

Two Major Types of Diabetes

	TYPE I INSULIN-DEPENDENT	TYPE II NON-INSULIN-DEPENDENT
Age at onset	Usually under 40, known as juvenile-onset diabetes	Usually over 40, known as maturity-onset diabetes
Prevalence	Less than 10 percent of all diabetics — about one million Americans	Greater than 90 percent of all diabetics — about 10 million Americans
Family history of diabetes	Occasionally	Common
Obesity at onset	Uncommon	Common If you are over 40 and at risk of getting diabetes (with a family history of it), being overweight will increase your risk. For tips on how to control your weight, see pages 130-131.
Symptoms at onset	Abrupt and severe (see facing page for symptoms)	Slower to occur and usually milder
Treatment	Daily insulin injections under strict medical supervision	Diet and exercise Studies show that overweight diabetics can bring their blood sugar levels down or back to normal by losing weight. See pages 84-85 for starting an exercise program and pages 130-131 for tips on weight control. (If diet and exercise are not successful, drugs may be required.)

Hypertension

SYSTOLIC (with diastolic 90 or less)	
Reading	Classification
139 or less	Normal
140 to 159	Borderline isolated systolic hypertension
160 or higher	Isolated systolic hypertension*

DIASTOLIC	
Reading	Classification
84 or less	Normal
85 to 89	High normal
90 to 104	Mild hypertension
105 to 114	Moderate hypertension
115 or higher	Severe hypertension

*Isolated systolic hypertension, when the systolic reading alone is elevated, is a common form of hypertension among the elderly.

Hypertension is known as "the silent killer" because it can develop and progress for years without producing symptoms. Unfortunately, the first sign can be a heart attack, stroke or kidney failure. As many as 60 million Americans have high blood pressure, making it one of the nation's most serious health concerns.

Blood pressure is indicated by two numbers, each referring to how high in millimeters the pressure of the blood in your arteries can raise a column of mercury (Hg). The first number, the systolic pressure, represents the force of blood during a heartbeat. The second number, the diastolic, indicates the pressure between beats. Normal blood pressure is defined as a systolic figure below 140 mm Hg and diastolic below 85 mm Hg. The box (left) shows the range of various classifications of blood pressure.

The common misconception of a typical hypertensive is of an overweight, overwrought male workaholic. In fact, there are no typical hypertensives: The disease can affect people of all races and social backgrounds. However, certain groups are more at risk than others. Blacks and Asians in Western cultures are more susceptible than whites, but a family history of the disease predisposes you to it.

While there is no cure for hypertension, most people can be treated with antihypertensive drugs, which must be continued for life. If you stop taking your medicine, and you do nothing else to control your hypertension, your blood pressure will rise again. Now more than 10 million Americans take antihypertensive medication. Many experts credit anti-hypertensive drugs with contributing significantly to a 31 percent decline in fatal heart disease between 1970 and 1986.

Despite their effectiveness, drugs are not the answer for everyone with hypertension. Several studies have questioned their value in treating patients with mild cases, for example. In addition, some people experience unpleasant side effects such as lethargy, loss of sexual desire, mood changes, depression, nighmares and loss of mental acuity. Fifty to 80 percent of patients, in fact, find that the side effects are more troubling than their supposedly symptomless disease, and either cut back on their dosage of medication or stop taking it completely.

Clearly, the best option is to find ways to reduce high blood pressure so that drug therapy can be reduced or eliminated. Chief among these methods are weight control and curtailment of excessive alcohol consumption. Studies show that when people gain weight, their blood pressure usually increases; conversely, when they lose weight, their blood pressure decreases. Studies also indicate that alcohol consumption has a similarly direct and significant effect on blood pressure.

There are other ways to lower your blood pressure. Although reducing salt and sodium intake may have a different effect on various people, a massive study of more than 10,000 men and women, the lower the sodium intake among a population, the lower the incidence of hypertension. Exercise can also have a beneficial effect on blood pressure. The chart (opposite) shows what you can do to reduce your blood pressure and some of the factors that may raise it.

Factors You Can Change

Exercise

Effect Regular physical exercise may lower mildly elevated blood pressure. Exercise also strengthens the cardiovascular system and reduces the risk of heart disease.

Recommendation Most experts recommend aerobic exercise such as jogging or swimming for 20-30 minutes at least three times a week. See pages 84-85 for an explanation of aerobic exercises. People with hypertension should avoid performing isometric exercise, such as weight lifting, since it can temporarily raise blood pressure to dangerous levels.

Calcium

Effect Studies suggest that inadequate calcium intake may result in high blood pressure. Taking calcium may be beneficial in both treating and preventing hypertension.

Recommendation Hypertensives and people at risk of developing it should meet the RDA for calcium (800 milligrams a day for adults). Low-fat dairy products are the best sources of calcium, since they also provide potassium and magnesium, which may help to keep blood pressure down. Calcium supplements are not absorbed by the body as well as dietary sources.

Relaxation techniques

Effect Meditation, hypnosis, biofeedback training and other relaxation techniques may produce a temporary reduction in blood pressure in some people. However, these techniques usually are not reliable or predictable enough to be considered effective treatments.

Recommendation Relaxation techniques should not be regarded as a first-line treatment for hypertension, but they may be useful as an adjunct to drug therapy in some circumstances.

Potassium

Effect Adequate potassium intake may help prevent or lower high blood pressure.

Recommendation If you eat a balanced diet, you most likely get enough potassium, since it is abundant in many foods. Orange juice, bananas, potatoes, dried fruit such as dates and figs, peanut butter, coffee and meat are especially good sources. By cutting down on high-sodium processed foods and substituting whole grains and fresh fruits and vegetables, you'll probably consume more potassium. Avoid supplements unless recommended by your doctor.

Sodium

Effect Numerous studies have found that people with high-sodium intake tend to have a high incidence of hypertension. People who reduce their sodium intake are likely to make other dietary changes that may lower blood pressure. While only 5 to 10 percent of the population is genetically sodium sensitive—that is, their blood pressure responds to the amount of sodium they consume—this group accounts for half the cases of hypertension in the United States.

Recommendation Because there is no practical way to determine who is sodium sensitive until hypertension develops, try to limit your sodium intake to no more than 2,000 to 3,000 milligrams per day (Americans typically consume two to three times as much.) Avoid processed and canned foods high in sodium. Do not use salt at the table and add no salt when you cook.

Overweight

Effect Obesity is a factor in 60 percent of all high blood pressure cases. Obese (20 percent or more above ideal weight) individuals are twice as likely to have high blood pressure as others.

Recommendation Even small weight reductions in obese people with hypertension can significantly lower blood pressure. For weight control tips, see pages 130-131.

Alcohol

Effect Excessive alcohol consumption is one of the most common causes of hypertension in the United States. Its effect on blood pressure appears to be completely reversible.

Recommendation Limit alcohol intake to two ounces a day. To help cut down on alcohol, see pages 52-53.

Type-A personality

Effect People with type-A personalities are susceptible to "labile" hypertension—erratic blood pressure—but it is not known whether such readings eventually lead to hypertension.

Recommendation Individuals with labile hypertension should be monitored by their doctors.

Cigarettes

Effect Smoking causes blood pressure to rise briefly, but its long-term effect is not clear.

Recommendation Smoking increases the risk of heart attack, and so does hypertension, so if you are a hypertensive smoker, the risks are compounded. For tips on how to quit smoking, see pages 118-119.

Caffeine

Effect Caffeine elevates blood pressure briefly, but its long-term effect is not known. Habitual users may develop some tolerance to its effects.

Recommendation Avoid caffeine one hour before having your blood pressure taken.

Stress

Effect Stress can raise blood pressure temporarily, but its long-term effect is not clear.

Recommendation A recent study of air-traffic controllers found that stress can lead to increased alcohol consumption, resulting in hypertension. For tips on how to relax, see pages 122-123.

Infectious Diseases

Infectious diseases are illnesses caused by various microorganisms commonly known as germs. These illnesses range from the deadly, such as AIDS and botulism, to the mundane, like the common cold. Two types of germs — pathogenic bacteria and viruses — are responsible for the majority of infectious diseases, although there are four other categories of germs that can result in illness: fungi, parasitic worms, protozoa and rickettsiae.

Infectious diseases are transmitted in a variety of ways that allow germs to invade your body through your skin, nose, mouth or other openings. Most respiratory ailments enter your body through your nose and throat. A study found that about 2 million viral particles are expelled when you sneeze, and about 91,000 are emitted when you cough.

Dysentery, trichinosis and botulism are transmitted via infected food or water. Cuts and small scratches in the skin provide entry for some infections, such as tetanus. Insect and animal bites are common modes of transmission of many serious illnesses, like Lyme disease and rabies. Sexually transmitted diseases (STDs), such as herpes, syphilis, gonorrhea and AIDS, result from germs passed via sexual contact.

With the prevalence of so many germs, it is surprising that humans do not contract more infections than they do. Blood clotting provides skin protection by rapidly closing wounds that might allow entry for some germs. Bodily secretions — such as mucus in your nose and throat, tears, saliva and stomach acid — protect against various other germs. Diligent personal hygiene can greatly reduce the number of germs that reach you.

If germs get through your body's primary defenses, your immune system combats them. This process involves both the circulatory and the lymphatic systems. When an invader enters the bloodstream, the lymph nodes increase the production of white blood cells, which might cause your glands to swell, and the cells engulf the germs. Invading germs can also precipitate fever, which destroys many heat-susceptible germs and slows their growth.

The immune system also produces antibodies specifically designed to destroy a particular germ. Antibodies function in a variety of ways: Some break germs apart, others inhibit their growth and a third type neutralizes their toxins. The formation of antibodies against a particular disease provides protection against repeat infections by the same germ. See the illustration (opposite) for how your body fights infection.

For some illnesses, antibiotics can help your body fight infection by destroying germs or increasing the effectiveness of your immune response. Immunization helps protect against disease by one of two ways: introducing into the blood a dead or weakened germ, such as the polio virus, which allows your body to build sufficient antibodies to resist it; or by introducing antibodies for a disease, such as rabies, produced by another person or animal.

A growing body of evidence indicates that you can improve your immune response to infection by adopting healthy lifestyle habits. For more information on how to fight infections, see common colds, pages 66-67; immunization, pages 100-101; over-the-counter drugs, pages 106-107; safe sex, pages 112-113.

How the Body Combats Infection

- **BONE MARROW** is a soft material that fills the cavities of bones and produces many of the white blood cells that eventually relocate to the spleen, lymph nodes and other lymphoid aggregations.

- **DIGESTIVE SYSTEM** contains glands that line the stomach wall and secrete hydrochloric acid, which destroys the majority of bacteria that enter the stomach with food. Some bacteria successfully survive the stomach's acid and relocate to the intestinal tract. The colon, part of the large intestine, is populated with normal bacteria that cause no harm.

- **LACHRYMAL GLANDS** in the upper outside region of each eye socket continually produce tears, which contain an antibacterial substance known as lysozyme. Tears also help to cleanse eyes by flushing out foreign particles.

- **LIVER** is a powerful detoxifying organ, capable of breaking down many types of toxic substances and making them less harmful. It also produces the components for blood clot formation.

- **LYMPHATIC SYSTEM** plays a crucial role in the body's defenses against disease. It acts as a second circulatory network, intertwined with the vascular circulation of the blood. Lymph, a tissue fluid that is transported by lymphatic vessels, contains white blood cells known as lymphocytes, which destroy bacteria and other foreign particles. Lymph nodes are situated along the lymphatic vessels. They manufacture lymphocytes and produce antibodies, which attack foreign substances. The nodes also trap bacteria and minute foreign particles. When fighting infection, they often swell in the neck, armpits and groin.

- **MUCOUS MEMBRANES** line the walls of body passages and cavities, such as the stomach and nose. The secreted mucous coats the membranes' surfaces and protects them from foreign substances that enter the body.

- **SALIVARY GLANDS** are situated under the tongue, in the cheeks and below the jaw. They secrete saliva, which contains leukocytes and elements of blood plasma that help to destroy bacteria, including the oral bacteria responsible for dental cavities.

- **SKIN** is first in line in the body's defense against infection. It is equipped with minute structures and mechanisms that prevent entrance of bacteria and other

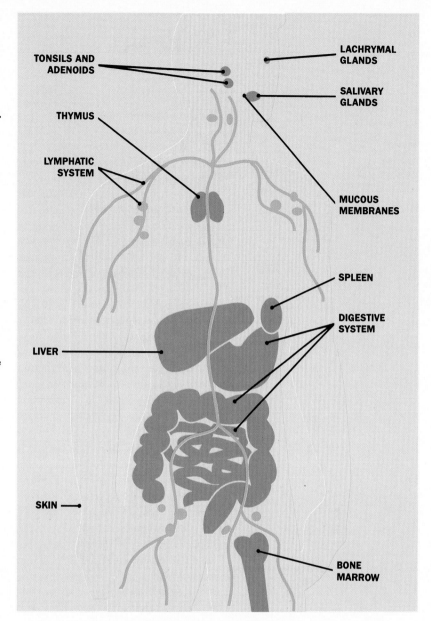

potentially harmful matter from the environment. And, because it is constantly renewing itself and casting off dead cells, foreign matter is rarely able to survive on the skin's surface.

- **SPLEEN** manufactures new lymphocytes, the white blood cells that help to defend the body against invading microorganisms. The spleen also contains many phagocytic cells that function as a cleansing system for the blood. These cells quickly remove infectious agents such as bacteria, parasites and debris from the blood. The spleen is an important supplier of antibodies, which help the body fight infection.

- **THYMUS** is situated in the upper part of the chest cavity. It is a temporary, lymphoid organ that is relatively large in infants, and develops until puberty, when it begins to gradually dwindle. Early in life, the thymus produces lymphocytes and sends them out to the spleen and the lymph nodes.

- **TONSILS** and **ADENOIDS** make up a band of lymphoid tissue at the throat. They are part of the lymphatic system, a protective group of cells that destroy bacteria. Their main function is to form antibodies against invading microorganisms that try to enter the respiratory and digestive tracts.

Stress

Although most people do not recognize stress as a direct cause of illness or mortality, the American Academy of Family Physicians estimates that about 66 percent of all visits to family doctors are prompted by stress-related disorders. Stress also contributes to coronary artery and lung disease, hypertension, cancer, accidents, cirrhosis of the liver and suicide. The annual costs of absenteeism, lost productivity and medical care as a result of stress are estimated to be $50 to $75 billion a year.

Almost 40 years ago, University of Washington psychiatrist Thomas Holmes and his colleague Richard Rahe observed that disruptive incidents, such as a death in the family or the loss of a job, often preceded the onset of disease among tuberculosis patients. Other research showed that samples of hospitalized patients — regardless of the nature of their illnesses — had significantly more serious and frequent stressful events, as measured on the Holmes-Rahe Social Readjustment Scale, than similar samples of people who were not in the hospital. *(See the chart opposite.)*

More recently, studies have shown that changes do not have to be major to impose stress and encourage illness. Researchers at the University of California, Berkeley, have determined that the cumulative effect of life's minor hassles — housework, deadline pressures and irritating noise, for example — can have an even greater effect. One study found that people who were subjected daily to the noise of air traffic near an airport were treated more often for hypertension and other stress-related disorders than those who lived in low-noise areas.

Numerous studies also show that hypertension and other illnesses seem to be associated with high-demand, low-control occupations. For instance, a study of Bay Area Rapid Transit (BART) bus drivers in the San Francisco area revealed that levels of hypertension and illness were highest among those who had been employed the longest, driving through San Francisco's congested streets, while struggling to adhere to impossible schedules.

Psychologists have recognized that how you deal with and confront life's stresses determines in large part how successfully you can triumph over them. Researchers Suzanne Kobasa and Salvatore R. Maddi, for instance, conducted a study of how the middle- and upper-level executives of Illinois Bell responded to the uncertainty of a court-ordered breakup of the corporation. As predicted by the Holmes-Rahe Social Readjustment Scale, some executives felt overwhelmed by the corporate upheavals and became ill. Other executives were less likely to become ill and reported sick about half as much as those who felt the strain. Kobasa and Maddi studied these "hardy" executives and found three of the following common characteristics in all of them:

CHALLENGE. Hardy executives saw change as a challenge, rather than a threat; it was an opportunity to try new and exciting ideas.

COMMITMENT. Hardy executives had a strong sense of purpose: They believed in themselves, their values and what they were doing in their careers.

CONTROL. They felt they had an influence on their lives. Rather than hope for good luck and wait for oth-

How Much Stress is Stress?

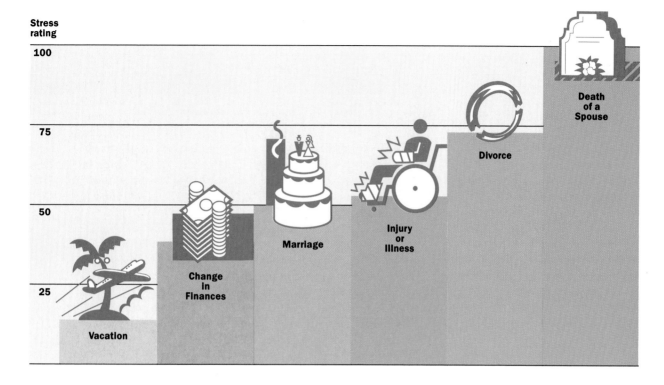

Stress rating

100

75

50

25

Vacation

Change in Finances

Marriage

Injury or Illness

Divorce

Death of a Spouse

ers to make decisions, they took initiative and made positive things happen as a result.

Most of the hardy executives reported that they were not born with the ability to confront stress successfully. They learned how to cope, and, indeed, many of them practiced coping behaviors and thoughts. Accepting change as a challenge rather than a threat is one way to cope with stress. When you can recognize such symptoms as foot tapping, clenched teeth and headaches, for example, you can reduce your stress level deliberately. One method is through relaxation techniques such as deep-breathing exercises, Yoga and meditation.

As part of the Medical Research Council (MRC) of Great Britain's five-year study of more than 17,000 men and women with mild hypertension, it was found that after one year,

patients who received relaxation and biofeedback training were able to stop taking antihypertensive drugs, yet maintain a safe blood pressure.

Exercise tends to reduce the perception of stress. Many people who perform aerobic exercise regularly report a calming effect that persists for two to five hours after a workout. Psychologists believe that regular exercise can improve your self-esteem and self-confidence and minimize any psychological feeling of impending doom. Studies have shown that physically active individuals tend to be at lower risk for hypertension, coronary artery disease, anxiety and other stress-related illnesses than sedentary people.

For information on stress management, see pages 122-123. See pages 48-49 for maintaining an active lifestyle and pages 84-85 for starting an exercise program.

In a famous study, people who reported the most stress in their lives — either positive or negative changes — seemed to suffer the most illnesses. Based on interviews with more than 5,000 subjects, researchers Thomas Holmes and Richard Rahe assigned numerical values to 43 events that tend to cause stress, and devised the Social Readjustment Scale. Those who scored more than 300 points had an 80 percent chance of becoming involved in accidents, developing ulcers, psychiatric disturbances or other serious illnesses within six months.

Stroke

Stroke, which afflicts a half-million Americans annually, is the third-leading cause of death in the United States, claiming more than 150,000 lives each year. Although most stroke victims survive a first attack, many are left handicapped: More than 2 million Americans are disabled by stroke.

A stroke is the result of a sudden disruption in blood supply to a part of the brain; if the supply is not restored, the brain cells die, and the victim loses certain functions. Common symptoms of stroke are paralysis of one side of the body, speech and vision impairment, confusion and temporary personality changes.

Fortunately, much of the neurological damage is reversible. When therapy is begun within 24 hours, healthy brain cells can quickly learn to perform the functions of damaged cells, allowing many victims to experience significant recovery.

According to the National Institute of Neurological and Communicative Disorders and Stroke, only one in 10 victims of hemiplegia is disabled permanently. One-half of stroke victims remain only partly handicapped and one-third recover fully. And the younger the victim, the greater the chance for recovery.

There are three basic types of stroke. The most common, a cerebral thrombosis, develops in a way identical to the coronary artery blockage that causes a heart attack: Deposits of fat and cholesterol block circulation to a part of the brain. In an embolic stroke, a blood clot becomes wedged in a cerebral artery. The vast majority of strokes — 70 to 80 percent — are either thrombotic or embolic. Less common, but occurring with higher fatality rates, are hemorrhagic strokes, which occur when an artery inside or on the surface of the brain bursts.

The death rate from stroke has dropped about 5.7 percent annually since 1973. Improved medical care is partly responsible for this significant decrease as well as recognizing the risk factors and early symptoms that signal the onset of stroke.

If you have a history of stroke in your family, or suffer from heart disease or diabetes, your risk is higher than others. Men have 30 percent more strokes than women; blacks are 60 percent more likely to have

Warning Signs of Stroke

A stroke results from damage to the brain tissue, usually because of a restricted or blocked artery that interrupts the supply of blood to the brain, or from a cerebral hemorrhage. Since each artery in the brain nourishes a specific part, the damage depends on which arteries and brain areas are affected. For instance, if there is tissue damage in the back area of the cerebral cortex, the section of the brain that controls visual function, vision is affected. Because a stroke can affect one or more areas of the brain, it is possible to have any of the following symptoms listed below.

- Sudden weakness or numbness in an arm, leg or facial muscles, usually only on one side of the body
- Difficulty in speaking or understanding speech
- Impaired vision, especially in one eye
- Dizziness or fainting, frequently accompanied by double vision
- Loss of balance or unsteadiness
- Headaches
- Abrupt personality disturbances such as impatience, irritability or suspiciousness
- Sudden hearing loss or ringing in ears
- Difficulty in swallowing
- Altered judgment or forgetfulness

strokes than whites. Although your risk more than doubles with each decade after age 55, strokes can occur at any age.

Four of five stroke victims have a history of ministrokes, which are known as transitory ischemic attacks (TIAs). Recognizable by brief dizziness, confusion or weakness, a TIA is caused by a momentary lack of oxygen in a small area of brain tissue. Consult a physician if you experience the symptoms of stroke or TIA.

You can further reduce your risk by modifying your lifestyle. Because stroke and heart disease are rooted in the same circulatory-related malfunctions, stroke prevention also benefits your heart by reducing the buildup of plaque in the arteries leading to your heart and brain.

High blood pressure, affecting more than half of stroke victims, is the greatest single contributor to stroke. Further, a high-fat diet develops fat deposits in your arteries.

Eating correctly, coupled with regular aerobic exercise, which improves circulation efficiency and raises the level of plaque-reducing HDL cholesterol, and weight control will help alleviate both risk factors. Because it may raise your blood pressure or affect circulation, stress is a secondary contributing factor to stroke; reducing stress may also help lessen hypertension.

Smoking also greatly increases your stroke risk. A recent 26-year longitudinal study of 4,000 subjects found that stroke risk increased with the number of cigarettes smoked.

Other research showed that men who were heavy smokers had three times as many strokes as nonsmokers. Another study determined that women who smoke less than a half pack a day more than doubled their risk of stroke.

Finally, there is evidence that oral contraceptives, especially when taken by women in their forties or who smoke, increase the risk of stroke. If you are in this category, or have other risk factors, evaluate your method of contraception.

For facts about birth control, see pages 62-63; cholesterol, pages 64-65; dietary fat, pages 80-81; fitness, pages 84-85; nutrition and diet, pages 104-105; smoking, pages 118-119; stress management, pages 122-123; weight control, pages 130-131.

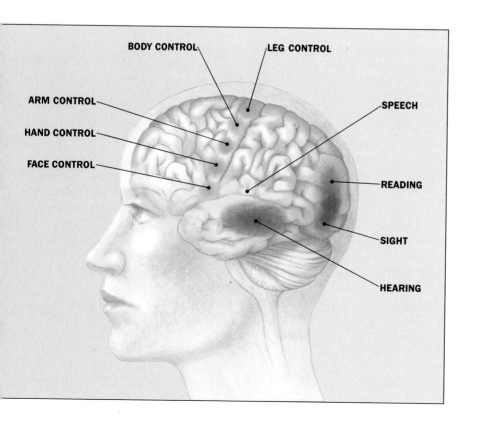

BODY CONTROL
LEG CONTROL
ARM CONTROL
SPEECH
HAND CONTROL
FACE CONTROL
READING
SIGHT
HEARING

Traumatic Injuries

Traumatic accidents — rapid or violent physical injuries — affect more than 10 million Americans each year and kill 100,000, making accidents the fourth-leading cause of death in this country. In children under 15, accidents are the primary cause of fatality, claiming 15,000 lives annually.

Automobile accidents, which account for almost 50 percent of all traumatic mishaps, lead the toll of accidental deaths among Americans under 65. Falls, more than half of which occur in the home, take second place overall, but are the leading cause of accidental death for those over 65. In order of frequency, drowning, burns, asphyxiation, choking, poisoning and gunshot wounds complete the list of fatal traumas.

However, unlike diseases, accidents are largely avoidable. By understanding the nature of accidents — where and when they occur, and what causes them — you can do much to prevent them.

Many automobile accidents could be avoided if proper safety restraints for both adults and children are used. According to one estimate, one-half of adult fatalities and 91 percent of the deaths of children under five could be prevented by the use of seat belts and child-restraint seats. The use of automobile air bags may further reduce the fatality rate.

Four million Americans are disabled in home accidents each year, and 27,000 are killed. Almost any sort of accident can occur at home, from burns, cuts, poisonings, electrical shocks and drownings to fatal falls. Most of them can be prevented if you eliminate hazards and practice home safety. Likewise, taking precautions during recreational activities also lessens the likelihood of drowning accidents, falls and gunshot wounds.

Research has shown that some occasions are more accident-prone than others. A study at the Boston Children's Hospital Medical Center found that more accidents occur between three and six in the afternoon — when the evening rush means that children are less supervised. Also, accidents happen more frequently when the family departs from its normal routine, even if only by being extra hungry or tired. More accidents occur on Saturdays than on any other day of the week.

Accident risks change for different age groups. Since falls take their greatest toll among the elderly, older people should take extra precautions. Although choking is the sixth-leading cause of fatality for children under six, it is the primary cause of accidental deaths in the home.

Studies show that people who are under stress tend to have mishaps frequently. If you are unhappy at your job or have troubles at home, for instance, you are more likely to be absentminded or careless and have accidents. It is important to recognize stress and learn to reduce its effects.

When accidents do occur, rapid responses can help save lives. Wounds, burns or fractures require immediate treatment, since they can also lead to shock, which can cause complications and death. Some of the symptoms of shock are depicted in the illustration *(right)*. Knowing first aid will help you to cope with injuries before medical care arrives.

For more information on preventing and treating traumatic injuries, see driving safety, pages 72-73; household safety, pages 98-99; stress management, pages 122-123; first-aid appendix, pages 136-141.

Shock: Signs and Symptoms

Shock can cause death from injuries or illnesses that would not normally be fatal. Shock may follow an accident, severe bleeding, heart attack, stroke, infection, extreme pain, broken bones, food or chemical poisoning, prolonged exposure to extreme cold or heat, excessive loss of body fluids as a result of vomiting or diarrhea or traumatic fear. Shock results when the circulatory system fails to provide sufficient blood to all parts of the body. If you can recognize the signs and symptoms listed below, you may be able to determine a victim's risk of going into shock and save his or her life. Have the person lie down, make sure he is warm, and raise his feet above his head. Call for medical assistance immediately.

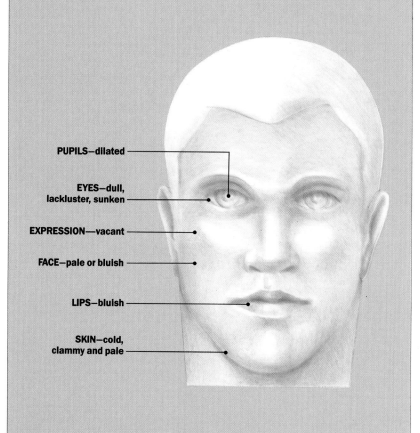

PUPILS—dilated

EYES—dull, lackluster, sunken

EXPRESSION—vacant

FACE—pale or bluish

LIPS—bluish

SKIN—cold, clammy and pale

ALSO LOOK FOR:

- Nausea or vomiting
- Extreme thirst
- Restlessness
- Anxiety
- Confusion
- Slurred speech
- Decreased body temperature
- Shallow and rapid breathing
- Trembling
- Unconsciousness
- Decreased blood pressure
- Weak and rapid pulse

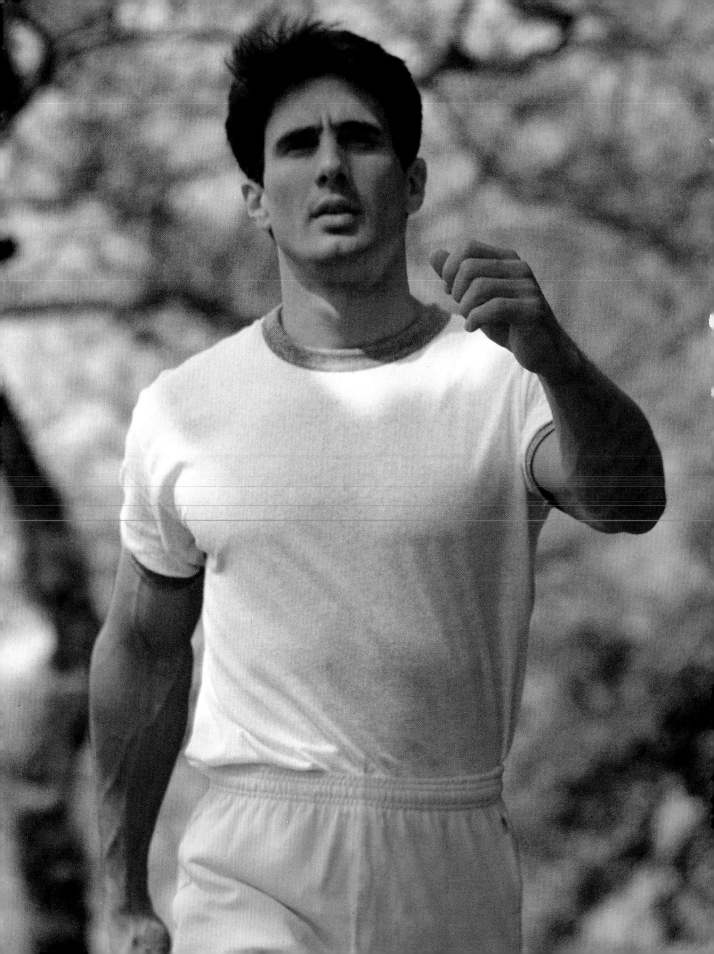

CHAPTER THREE

Staying Well

A practical guide

T his section, which is the largest in the book, presents essential and useful information on a multitude of topics that constitute wellness. The topics are arranged in alphabetical order for easy reference, and, in each case, an explanation is accompanied with practical tips and guidelines. If you have taken the Health-Risk-Assessment Questionnaire and read the material about health risks in the previous chapter, you should have a sense of which topics are most relevant to you. As you look through the section, additional topics may interest you, and you can also increase your knowledge about the factors that contribute to a healthy lifestyle.

The recommendations on the following pages take into account the latest findings in the fields of preventive health care, nutrition and exercise. The intent, though, is not simply to be current, but to provide information that is both practical and also likely to be upheld over time. For example, scientists may continue to quibble about the details of how plaque forms in coronary arteries. But there is little argument that a diet high in saturated fats and cholesterol contributes to plaque formation, and that you can very likely reduce your risk of heart disease by limiting fat and cholesterol in your diet. Beyond that, it helps to know which types of food are highest in fat, and if all fatty foods are equally bad for you (they are not). Recognizing that information in health is subject to revision, the guidelines presented here are backed by the consensus of experts as well as studies showing their value and effectiveness at improving health.

Of all the elements of wellness, nutrition is foremost, and a number of the topics are devoted to nutritional concerns. One of the ironies of modern life is that while Americans are living longer than they did at the turn of the century, many of the foods they eat have declined in quality. Food-processing techniques remove fiber and nutrients while infusing foods with preservatives, sugar, sodium and fat, contributing to obesity and many other health problems that limit longevity. Despite the prevalence of processed foods, it is important to remember that there is still a wide selection of nutritious foods available. In the following pages, you will find topics such as Cholesterol, Fats, Fiber, Vitamins and Minerals and Weight Control, as well as material on how to make wise choices in restaurants and how to interpret the confusing information on ingredients lists (see Eating Out and Food Labels).

Two other vital components of wellness are exercise and stress management. Several long-term studies that compare the lifestyles of thousands of individuals over decades have shown that regular exercise and an active lifestyle not only reduce the incidence of numerous chronic diseases, but slow many of the effects of aging. In addition, people who remain physically active are less prone to depression and have more self-confidence than those who are sedentary. Perhaps it is because they feel more in control of their lives, or possibly because activity and exercise encourage the release of chemical neurotransmitters in the brain that affect mental states. Whatever the reason, the daily stresses of life often seem more manageable to those who are active. Researchers have also uncovered methods to cope with job-related stress and emotional problems. Three topics — Active Lifestyle, Fitness and Stress Management — offer guidelines for reducing stress.

Environmental factors are increasingly becoming crucial elements of maintaining optimal health. While industrial pollution may pose serious health risks, people may be less aware that common household contaminants pose a greater cancer risk to the public. Fortunately, you can take steps to reduce those risks. The procedures outlined in Home Environment will help you determine if there are any toxic substances in your home, and tell how to remove them or minimize their risk. Outside the home, some researchers contend that a leading environmental risk stems from atmospheric pollution that is depleting the ozone layer and allowing more harmful ultraviolet radiation to reach the earth. Excessive exposure to the sun is known to be a factor in causing skin cancer; in the United States, there are 400,000 cases each year. You can reduce your risk of this form of cancer by following the simple precautions in Sun Safety.

In emphasizing preventive health measures, wellness does not imply that you should avoid medical advice and treatment when needed; ideally, you are in a partnership with your doctor to avert illness. The information in Doctors includes advice on how to find the best primary-care physician for your medical needs. In addition, the chart on page 103 indicates how often you should have routine checkups and specific tests according to your sex and age. Since early detection of cancer is your best chance for cure, you should not only visit your doctor, but also perform self-examinations regularly. In the case of breast cancer, for example, the American Cancer Society estimates that about 90 percent of all early detections are found not by a physician, but by the woman herself or her sexual partner. For tips on how to perform these exams, see Medical Self-Tests.

Other topics are more specialized, though still relevant to millions of people. For instance, the information in Alcoholism and Smoking covers two of the most serious, preventable health problems in the United States. Research has shown that while both alcohol and nicotine are powerfully addictive drugs, they can be overcome. Many individuals who smoke or who drink alcohol excessively want to give up these habits, but feel powerless to do so, especially if they have tried and failed. While giving up any addiction is often difficult, some methods have been proven to work better than others. For example, despite the advertising claims of many smoking-cessation programs that urge tapering off slowly, surveys show that quitting all at once is your best chance of giving up cigarettes permanently.

Along with showing you how to reduce health risks, this chapter can help you with smaller concerns that contribute to your well-being. For example, to learn some reasons for sleeping problems, along with helpful hints on getting a good night's rest, see the section titled Sleep. Four out of five adults have foot problems, and about the same proportion suffer backaches — yet much of this discomfort can be easily prevented, as explained in Foot Care and Back Pain. You will also find self-care measures for such common complaints as allergies, arthritis, asthma, colds, headaches, sports injuries and other ailments.

Despite the diversity and number of the topics in this section, maintaining a healthy lifestyle need not involve radical changes or sacrifices. Indeed, a radical change can backfire. For example, many people embark on a vigorous exercise program with great enthusiasm, only to drop out after a few days or weeks because of injuries or boredom. The box on page 85 gives you a simple formula for starting an exercise program gradually, so that you can avoid injury and get used to including exercise as part of your daily routine. Similarly, many of the guidelines throughout this chapter consist of quick, easy steps that make wellness manageable.

What are the hidden costs of smoking? According to a study by researchers at the University of Michigan and the RAND Corporation, the total population pays higher insurance rates — whether or not people smoke — to cover smokers' medical bills. This amounts to about 38 cents for each pack of cigarettes. However, since smokers die an average of 137 minutes per pack sooner than nonsmokers, they are not alive to use as much public and private pensions as nonsmokers. All totaled, smokers save society about 91 cents per pack of cigarettes.

Active Lifestyle

According to the Harvard Alumni Study illustrated on the facing page, those who expended 2,000 or more calories a week had the greatest increase in longevity. To burn 2,000 calories a week, you would have to exercise for about 30 minutes five days a week. If you did that for 20 years, for every hour of exercise, you would gain almost seven hours in longevity.

Medical science has improved our lives and increased our longevity. Modern antibiotics, new methods for fighting cancer and the benefits of good nutrition have not only added years to our lives, but made them more comfortable and pain free. It is also accepted that avoiding harmful habits, such as cigarette smoking and drug abuse, can ensure a longer and more enjoyable life. However, you should do more than avoid harmful substances and be the passive recipient of good medical care — you should stay active physically.

Several recent large-scale studies have shown that you can improve your well-being and longevity by leading an active lifestyle, which means performing a regular exercise program and engaging in active pursuits. These studies show that people who remain active and physically fit tend to live longer, healthier lives and be less prone to depression, anxiety and stress than sedentary individuals. In addition, active people are more likely to report that they feel invigorated, happy and sleep more soundly than others who do not exercise regularly.

In the Aerobics Center Longitudinal Study, which followed more than 10,000 men over eight years and related their exercise and activity habits with overall mortality, researchers found that both physical activity and fitness were independently associated with increased longevity. Other studies have suggested that you can improve your longevity with moderate physical activity such as walking, climbing stairs, gardening and taking weekend hikes.

How much longer can you expect to live by staying active? In an ongoing study, which has been underway for more than 25 years, Dr. Ralph S. Paffenbarger Jr. and his associates at Stanford University are examining the lifestyles of nearly 17,000 Harvard alumni who entered college between 1916 and 1950. The study charts the lifestyles, health and mortality of the graduates when they were in school, during their middle age, and as they get older. The researchers are compiling and analyzing all of the subjects' social habits, physical activities and family histories of disease as well as data on such factors as mental illness, suicide, accidental death, cardiovascular disease and cancer. The findings have been published in a number of papers that show that subjects who exercised and remained active throughout their lives tended to live longer than their sedentary peers.

According to the study, an active lifestyle confers an average of one to two or more years of life (see the chart opposite). Although two years may not seem like much when you consider a lifetime of 70 years or more, it is the equivalent of the average extension of life if all forms of cancer were eliminated.

There are other reasons for being fit. The Harvard study and a number of others have shown that regular exercise is associated with lower blood cholesterol levels and reduced risk of cardiovascular disease. Active individuals are less at risk than sedentary people for other illnesses such as heart attack, hypertension, stroke, respiratory disease, osteoporosis and some forms of cancer.

If you want to lose weight, or if you are trying to maintain your current weight, physical activity and regular exercise are the best ways to do it, especially if you also restrict your calorie intake. Dieting by itself has been shown to reduce lean muscle tissue, rather than strictly fat tissue.

Activity and Longevity

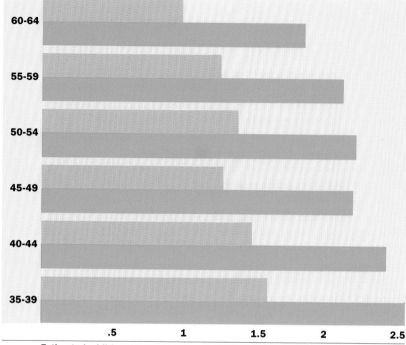

Age at beginning of study

60-64	
55-59	
50-54	
45-49	
40-44	
35-39	

.5　　1　　1.5　　2　　2.5

Estimated additional years to life

▢ Vigorous sports with varied caloric expenditure
▢ Activities known to expend 2,000 or more calories per week

Also, just dieting is notorious for achieving short-term weight loss, leading to a gradual return to your previous weight. Staying active is one of the best ways to ensure that you lose weight on a long-term basis. Regular exercise also ensures that you retain muscle tissue.

Despite the benefits of an active lifestyle, unfortunately, most Americans remain sedentary. The United States Public Health Service estimates that 80 percent of the population is either completely sedentary or exercises at an intensity too low or too infrequently to derive any fitness or health benefit. So serious is the problem that the Institute of Medicine has concluded that lifestyle habits, including lack of exercise, result in the heaviest burden of illness in the United States.

If you wish to begin a program of regular exercise, it is important to choose activities that you enjoy, preferably ones that involve family members or friends. Studies show that you are also more likely to continue with activities that are accessible, inexpensive and challenging, such as bike trips, canoeing, walking, hiking, running, swimming, aerobic dance and cross-country skiing.

Start exercising slowly to avoid injury and increase the chance that you will stay with your program. Increase the intensity or duration of your workout by no more than 10 percent. For tips on beginning an exercise program, see pages 84-85.

An active lifestyle may add years to your life. In a study of almost 17,000 Harvard alumni, researchers compared three groups: 1. sedentary people who played no vigorous sports, expending less than 500 calories per week on physical activity; 2. moderately active individuals who regularly engaged in vigorous sports such as tennis or soccer; and 3. people who expended 2,000 or more calories a week in sports, exercise and other activities. The chart above shows the average additional longevity of the two active groups compared with their sedentary peers.

Aging and Fitness

Researchers at Loma Linda University Human Performance Laboratory tested the 78-year-old record holder of the marathon for all women over 65. This woman, who began running at age 63 and completed her first marathon when she was 70, was found to have the aerobic capacity of college women who were not in the habit of training. The marathon runner had, in effect, turned back her aerobic clock by almost 60 years.

As Americans grow older, researchers have become more interested in the process of aging, the special requirements of older people, and the factors that cause some individuals to age quickly while others live a long and vigorous life with few health problems.

Some of the findings have been surprising: Many of the symptoms that we associate with aging, such as weight gain, decreased muscle tone and flexibility, diminished aerobic capacity, bone mineral loss, a slowing down of reflexes and depression, are not the inevitable results of growing older; they are more often symptoms of inactivity.

Much of the research on exercise and aging has centered on aerobic capacity, as determined by your VO_2max, or the measurement of the maximum capacity of your heart, lungs and muscles to transport and utilize oxygen. Your VO_2max normally declines by about one percent each year past the age of 30. However, with aerobic endurance training, middle-aged and elderly people can reclaim their aerobic capacity of 20 years earlier; well-conditioned individuals in their 60s and 70s often display the aerobic capacity of younger sedentary people in their 20s. No drug can offer such promise for health and vigor as a regular program of exercise that includes aerobic activities.

It is never too late to improve your fitness. In a study of men aged 49 to 65 who embarked on a 30- to 45-minute-per-day walking and jogging program three days per week, researchers found that the men improved their average VO_2max by 18 percent after 20 weeks of training. With just five months of moderate aerobic training, the majority of these men were able to improve their condition significantly.

Besides improving your cardiorespiratory fitness and increasing lean body mass and muscle endurance, exercise may also help lower your blood pressure and cholesterol levels, which tend to rise with age, reduce stress and aid in weight control. Exercise also minimizes the tendency among older people to faint or loose their balance. In addition, weight-bearing activities like brisk walking may help delay or prevent the development of osteoporosis.

If you are currently exercising, you are probably taking the most effective step to stay vigorous and healthy. If you are sedentary and over 45, however, or if you smoke, have high blood pressure or have not exercised regularly for two years or more, you should consult your physician before you engage in strenuous exercise. Stop immediately if you feel any chest pain, dizziness or nausea. Also, avoid outdoor exercise in extreme heat or cold. Although you should expect minor aches and pains when you begin exercising, cut back if you feel discomfort.

The Council on Scientific Affairs recommends that you start with brisk walking. Cycling, swimming and running are all excellent forms of exercise. Running, however, because of the high-impact pounding of the running stride, may predispose older persons to bone and joint injuries if they are unaccustomed to it.

Although performing any amount of physical activity is better than none at all, you should aim for at least 20 minutes of sustained, vigorous exercise three times a week. The council also suggests that you can benefit from activities such as stair climbing and gardening. See pages 48-49 for the benefits of an active lifestyle and pages 84-85 for tips on starting a fitness program.

Slowing the Effects of Aging

BRAIN
As you age, nerve cells die and your memory starts to fade. Researchers have found that activities such as reading, writing, participating in stimulating conversations, creative endeavors and going to lectures, museums and the theater can help keep you alert and functioning at your best.

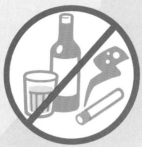

BLOOD PRESSURE
By age 70, your systolic blood pressure rises 10-40 points; diastolic blood pressure rises 5-10 points. Two important steps to lowering blood pressure: do not smoke an do not consume more than two alcoholic drinks a day. Also maintain an active lifestyle and engage in aerobic exercise at least three times a week.

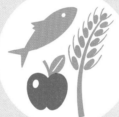

CARDIORESPIRATORY SYSTEM
Your heart's pumping capacity can diminish by 30 percent by the time you are 70; lung capacity can drop 50 percent. To maintain or improve your heart's ability to pump blood, engage in aerobic exercise regularly and maintain a nutritious low-fat, low-cholesterol diet.

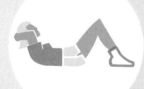

MUSCLES
Between 30-70 years, your muscle mass diminishes 25-30 percent and flexibility decreases 20-30 percent. To maintain muscle tone, build strength and improve your range of motion, engage in stretching and muscle-strengthening exercises, such as sit-ups and push-ups, regularly.

SKIN
Over time, your skin can become coarse, wrinkled and blotched. Minimize sun exposure as much as possible. Ultraviolet rays are responsible for many skin ailments associated with age. Experts agree that everyone, even people with extremely dark skin, is susceptible to premature skin aging caused by over-exposure to the sun.

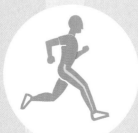

BONES
By age 70, bone density diminishes an average of 15-20 percent for men and 25-30 percent for women. Stay active, exercise and maintain proper nutrition. Do not smoke, and limit your intake of alcohol. To help slow osteoporosis, perform weight-bearing exercises at least three time a week, such as exercise walking, jogging and sit-ups.

Alcoholism

What are the costs of drinking alcohol? According to a study by researchers at the University of Michigan and the RAND Corporation, the medical and pension costs of each ounce of alcohol consumed per day in excess of two drinks is 63 cents. In addition, that same ounce of alcohol results in a loss of 20 minutes of the drinker's life.

Alcoholism is a complex, biological and psychological disorder that has a devastating impact on our nation's health and welfare. According to recent figures, alcohol causes or is associated with 200,000 deaths in the United States every year. This includes deaths directly attributable to alcohol-related diseases and traumatic events, such as automobile accidents and drownings. Indeed, half of all motor-vehicle-related deaths and half of all homicides can be attributed to alcohol abuse; one-quarter of all suicides have a likewise connection.

Alcohol is abused by approximately 10 million Americans. The annual costs of this abuse include $3.6 billion in property damage from motor-vehicle accidents, $3.1 billion in criminal-justice expenses, $507 million from fire losses and $54 million in social programs.

The wide-ranging effects of alcohol on your mind and body depends on a number of variables: your sex and body weight, how much you eat and the type of alcohol you drink over a time period. Unlike most other substances, alcohol is absorbed into your bloodstream from your stomach and small intestines, allowing it to affect your body quickly.

Five ounces of wine, 12 ounces of beer and 1.5 ounces of 80-proof liquor all put the same amount of alcohol into your blood — two-thirds of an ounce. Because they are less concentrated, beer and wine are absorbed more slowly than liquor. The carbon dioxide in champagne and in drinks mixed with soda increases alcohol absorption; eating while or before drinking slows it.

Once an ounce of alcohol is absorbed into your bloodstream, it takes your body about an hour to metabolize it. Thus, because alcohol is removed slowly from your blood, more than one drink per hour produces a steady increase in blood alcohol levels. All the cells in your body can absorb alcohol, so even its short-term use can have wide-ranging effects. Prominent among these are the effects of alcohol on your brain and central nervous system, causing progressive changes in judgment, memory and sensory perception.

Chronic, long-term alcohol abuse can seriously damage nearly every function and organ of your body. Your digestive system, particularly your liver, is overtaxed in metabolizing alcohol. Cirrhosis, irreversible liver damage attributed to an accumulation of fat associated with long-term drinking, occurs in about 15 percent of heavy drinkers and leads to severe complications and death. Alcoholics also are more likely to develop peptic ulcers and pancreatitis than nonalcoholics, and they often suffer from gastritis.

One of the worst effects of alcohol is on the nervous system, which can be temporarily or irreversibly damaged, perhaps even leading to psychosis. The cardiovascular system is also affected, resulting in increases in blood pressure and damage to the heart muscle. Consumption of alcohol during pregnancy can lead to serious physical and mental defects in the newborn.

While alcohol is not a carcinogen, excessive use of it, particularly in combination with tobacco, increases your chances of developing cancer of the mouth, larynx and throat. Alcohol abuse also appears to play a role in stomach and colon/rectal cancer and possibly in liver cancer.

Controlling Your Drinking

While the only certain way to avoid alcoholism is to abstain from drinking, many people can enjoy an occasional drink without becoming alcohol dependent. The following tips will help keep your social drinking within reasonable limits. If these measures are hard for you to adhere to, you might already have a drinking problem, and you should consult your physician or your local chapter of Alcoholics Anonymous.

◆ Measure your drinks so that you do not consume more alcohol than your body can metabolize in an hour. Two-thirds of an ounce of alcohol — equivalent to five ounces of wine, 12 ounces of beer or 1.5 ounces of liquor — is the maximum amount that a 160-pound man should have in one hour; a person who weighs less than that should drink less. Remember, do not drink alcohol on an empty stomach, since the alcohol is quickly absorbed into your body.

◆ You will probably drink less if you avoid holding a glass in your hand constantly. If you finish your drink in less than an hour, switch to a nonalcoholic beverage.

◆ Mix liquor or wine with plain water. If you are enjoying a glass of fine wine and do not want to dilute it, alternate sips of wine with water.

◆ Try mixed drinks without alcohol, such as a Bloody Mary without the vodka (also known as a Virgin Mary) or a Tom Collins without the gin.

◆ Make sure that the label on nonalcoholic beer includes the words "alcohol-free," since nonalcoholic beers may legally contain a small amount of it.

Fortunately, many of the serious physical consequences of alcoholism can be completely halted or reversed if drinking is discontinued. However, it can be difficult to determine that you have a drinking problem, and even more difficult to correct it. Even health-care professionals do not have a clear-cut definition of alcoholism, since not all heavy drinkers have dysfunctional lives.

The causes of alcoholism are poorly understood. Most people can drink occasionally and never succumb to alcohol abuse. Evidence indicates that there might be a genetic factor that predisposes people to it. Studies show that a significant number of children of alcoholic parents become alcoholics. Still, everyone with a hereditary tendency does not become an alcoholic, while many with nonalcoholic families are abusers.

Your best bet for avoiding alcohol abuse is not to drink it at all. If you do drink, however, do so in moderation, using the guidelines in the box *(above)*. And, while there is no standard definition of alcoholism, there are several signals of potential abuse. Seek help if you drink alcohol to relieve pain or stress, or have a pattern to control your drinking. Most experts agree that no alcoholic can ever learn to drink moderately; the only answer is to stop.

Finally, be aware that alcoholism can be treated successfully with professional or group help and the support of family and friends, although the desire to stop is probably the most critical factor. If you believe that you or a loved one has an alcohol problem, get help from Alcoholics Anonymous. A list of publications and free brochures are available from the General Service Office of Alcoholics Anonymous, P.O. Box 459, Grand Central Station, New York, NY 10163.

Allergies

More than 35 million Americans know that allergies are nothing to sneeze at. Their runny noses, sneezing, congestion and itchy eyes are unpleasant at best, and some allergic reactions can be fatal. But recent headway in immunology may relieve the symptoms of allergy sufferers.

The terms "hay fever" are misnomers, since hay does not cause the problem, nor does it result in fever. Instead, hay fever is usually an allergic response, to airborne pollen and mold spores; other allergens include animal dander, foods, feathers, cosmetics and certain drugs. Allergens may be inhaled, swallowed, rubbed on your skin or injected. Poison ivy is a common allergen that can cause intensely itchy or painful skin eruptions. Some people are allergic to penicillin or bee stings, both of which are occasionally fatal.

An allergic reaction is a complex immune response to substances in your body. Although a healthy immune system is crucial for fighting infections and viruses, an allergy is actually the result of a hypersensitivity of your immune system to a harmless substance.

An antibody called immunoglobulin E, or IgE, which is produced primarily in the lymph nodes and the mucous membranes of your nose and respiratory tract, attaches itself to allergens and also to immune defense cells called mast cells. Researchers observe that when the attachments are complete, these mast cells seem to explode literally, releasing histamine and other substances into the blood, causing tiny blood vessels to relax and exude fluids, resulting in swelling and itching in your eyes and nose. Histamine can also make breathing uncomfortable by causing your mucous glands to exude a thin mucus and by constricting your air passages.

Treatment for allergies has traditionally been to administer drugs that suppress or minimize the symptoms, such as antihistamines, which blunt the effect of the histamine released by the mast cells. Many of these drugs, however, have adverse side effects like drowsiness and mental dullness. Another way to combat allergies is to administer progressively increasing doses of an allergen in a series of injections to desensitize the patient. Many people with allergies simply opt to suffer.

Researchers believe that new drugs may soon effectively inhibit allergic responses. Immunologists have identified the structure of complex proteins that act as receptors on the surfaces of mast cells. These receptors are the attachment points for allergen-carrying immunoglobulin E. Now researchers feel confident that drugs can be developed to block them, thus preventing the mast cells from releasing histamines, which bring on the allergy symptoms.

The first step in preventing an allergic reaction is to find out what causes it. You may be able to determine this by noticing whether your symptoms occur in relation to a specific allergen. If you are unable to pinpoint the cause, however, consult an allergy specialist. Besides determining the source of your allergy, the specialist may also be able to prescribe drugs that will stop the production of histamines.

Once you identify the allergen that bothers you, how do you avoid it? If the problem is a cosmetic, feather pillow, household pet or food, the

Ragweed Density in the United States

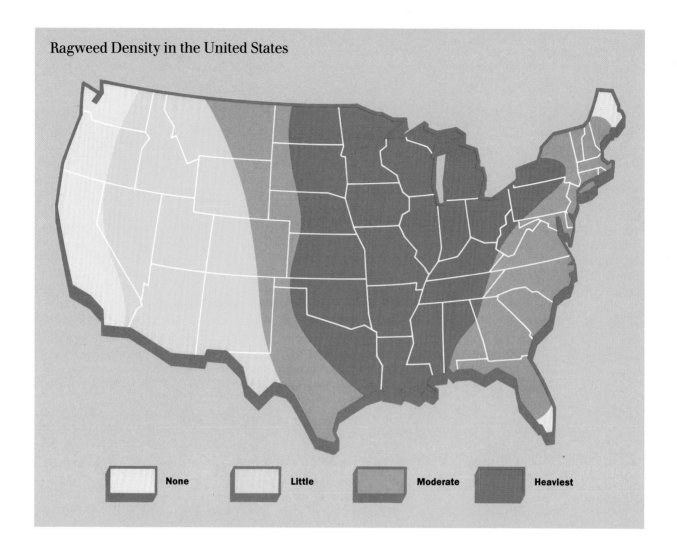

None   Little   Moderate   Heaviest

solution may be fairly simple. If you are allergic to ragweed, you might vacation in some region that is free of this plant during the ragweed season *(see the map above)*. Almost anyplace outside North America will do, except the western coast of France. The Pacific coast has almost no ragweed, but it does have other pollens. Arid regions may have less pollen, and you may also find relief at the seashore or any other area that does not have ragweed.

Many radio and television stations broadcast daily pollen counts during peak seasons, but these are of little practical value, since they are usually made the previous day from different locations, and may not be related to your symptoms.

Keep your windows closed during hay fever season and use an air conditioner, if you have one, to filter out as much pollen as possible. Drive your car with the windows closed. Do not hang sheets and clothing out to dry.

Pollen is likely to be worse in rural and suburban areas than in cities. Rain, however, can be a mixed blessing: A rainstorm will clean the air of pollen, but if rain is followed by several days of warm, windy weather, the pollen count will probably be higher than ever, and your symptoms will return.

Airborne pollen from ragweed is the major cause of hay fever in the United States. Because of the huge quantities of pollen released, even urban areas are susceptible to high pollen counts. Although ragweed is widespread throughout the country, little of it grows in areas that are dense with northern conifers, such as in the Pacific northwest or in Maine.

Arthritis

Arthritis is often called the great crippler. Indeed, more than 36 million Americans have it, but it does not necessarily mean an increasingly handicapped life. Most cases are managed easily and successfully, and with proper care and exercise, many people can live without pain and maintain good joint flexibility. Although the disease is incurable, arthritis remains treatable even in its most crippling and severe manifestations.

Arthritis, or joint inflammation, is a symptom of over 100 distinct but related illnesses referred to as rheumatic diseases. While joint inflammation is a symptom of them all, they can also affect the skin, muscles, connective tissues, tendons, ligaments and the protective coverings of some internal organs. The most common types of arthritis are osteoarthritis and rheumatoid arthritis, which is more severe. Other arthritic conditions and disorders include systemic lupus erythematosus, juvenile arthritis, gout, bursitis, tendinitis and ankylosing spondylitis. These rheumatic diseases all are chronic, lasting a long time or recurring many times. Most are incurable but remissions are common.

Osteoarthritis is usually the least severe rheumatic illness. About 90 percent of all people over 40 show some signs of osteoarthritis, although few of them have chronic disability or severe, degenerative joint disease. In osteoarthritis, cartilage, and sometimes bone, breaks down, possibly as the result of years of normal wear and tear on your joints. The joints most commonly affected are your fingers, hips, knees and spine.

Rheumatoid arthritis, the second most common rheumatic disease, can be much more serious. Unlike cases of osteoarthritis, rheumatoid arthritis often affects many joints simultaneously, often beginning in both hands and wrists or both feet. In addition, it is a systemic disease that can attack skin, muscles, blood vessels and, on occasion, the lungs and heart. Rheumatoid arthritis affects between one and three percent of the population, and is more than twice as likely to attack women as men. Although it can strike at any age, it usually begins between the ages of 40 and 60. Characteristically, the symptoms of rheumatoid arthritis conditions can change suddenly, either for the better or worse. Indeed, about 10 to 20 percent of all

Osteoarthritis of the finger joints can often be minimized with regular finger exercises. Perform the series of gentle stretching and strengthening exercises shown below.

Hand and Finger Exercises

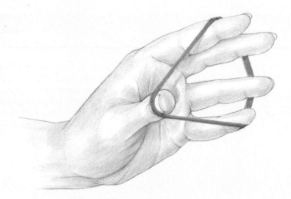

Place a large rubber band around your fingers. Open and close your hand against the resistance.

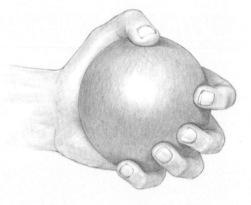

Hold a tennis ball, sponge or a piece of foam rubber in your palm. Squeeze your fingers around it, then release.

arthritis patients experience a complete remission.

The common denominator of all arthritic illness is joint pain due to a breakdown in the smooth functioning of joints. In normal joints, bone ends are covered by cartilage, which is a tough, flexible tissue that keeps bones from rubbing directly against one another. The joints are bathed in synovial fluid, which keeps them lubricated to ensure smooth and normal movement.

In arthritis, the joints become inflamed. Normally, inflammation serves a useful purpose in the process of protection and repair, usually by restricting movement so that the tissue has time to heal. Indeed, musculoskeletal pain and stiffness is a common symptom in virtually every disease known to man. However, in arthritis, the inflammatory process persists beyond the point of tissue repair. Chronic inflammation eventually leads to an erosion of synovial membrane, cartilage and bone.

Researchers believe that many cases of arthritis may be caused by a malfunction of the immune system, which sometimes attacks normal tissue as if it were hostile viruses, bacteria or cancer cells. What causes this inappropriate immune response is not clearly understood. In some cases, there seems to be a genetic factor that causes it. In others, an infection such as untreated gonorrhea, syphilis, chlamydia, viral hepatitis, rubella or Lyme disease may be the triggering agent.

Be alert to the warning signs of arthritis. You should see your physician so that he or she can make an accurate diagnosis if any of the following symptoms persist: early morning stiffness, swelling, recurring pain or tenderness in one or more joints, change in normal joint mobility, redness and warmth in a joint, and unexplained weight loss, fever or weakness in association with any manifestation of joint pain.

Short of maintaining your general good health, at this time, there are no effective, preventive measures you can take against arthritis. And while there is no real cure for the disease, early treatment and careful management allows most people with arthritis to maintain joint mobility.

Many people with osteoarthritis can maintain flexibility, and even restore it to some degree, through a well-designed exercise program that is implemented gradually and followed regularly. Indeed, the natural tendency to minimize the movement of arthritic joints will only lead to more stiffness and pain, since inactivity weakens the muscles that stabilize your joints.

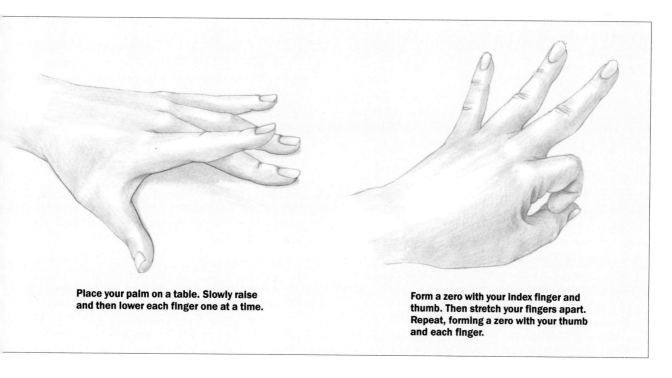

Place your palm on a table. Slowly raise and then lower each finger one at a time.

Form a zero with your index finger and thumb. Then stretch your fingers apart. Repeat, forming a zero with your thumb and each finger.

Asthma

Recent developments in the treatment of asthma have brought good news to the 9 million Americans who suffer from this chronic respiratory disease, which causes attacks of breathlessness, coughing and wheezing. Although asthma is incurable, new drug therapies can actually prevent attacks. Research showing the benefits of exercise is allowing asthmatics to enjoy active lives. In addition, those who suffer asthma attacks after exertion can learn to minimize their effects through simple breathing techniques or even by avoiding certain foods.

What is Asthma?

An asthma attack is an abnormal respiratory reaction to one or more irritants. It usually begins suddenly, and may be mild and transitory, or severe enough to require emergency treatment. In an attack, there is a constriction of the trachea and the connecting network of bronchial tubes. The smooth muscle surrounding the small bronchioles deep in the lungs goes into spasm, the membranes lining the bronchioles swell and secretions of mucus in the tubes increase. Air flow to and from the lungs is reduced, resulting in coughing, wheezing and a general shortness of breath.

An asthma attack makes it more difficult to exhale than inhale, which leads to a buildup of stale air in the air sacs, or alveoli, causing them to overstretch. Repeated attacks can damage the alveoli, which diminishes lung capacity and may eventually lead to emphysema or other pulmonary disorders. About 4,000 people die annually from asthma, and this number of cases has actually increased in recent years.

Who Gets Asthma?

Asthmatics are sensitive to a number of irritants that cause no respiratory distress in most people. In many cases, asthma is an allergic response. While a single, specific cause cannot always be found, common irritants are pollen, dust, animal hair and skin, feathers, mold spores, cigarette smoke, chemicals, flour, drugs and certain foods. Half of all asthmatics are children; attacks may become less frequent as a child grows.

Asthma can also occur at any age from such sources as respiratory infections, strenuous exercise or sudden exposure to cold air. In recent years, there has been a worldwide increase in the number of hospital admissions for asthma attacks in children under 14, which may be the result of air pollution.

While it has been speculated that asthma is emotionally induced, current research does not support this theory. An upset, however, might bring on an attack in someone who already has asthma.

How to Minimize the Effects of Asthma

An accurate diagnosis is an important first step to effective management. Determining just what triggers asthma in an individual is not always easy or possible, since there might be a whole constellation of irritants. If the triggers are known, the obvious step is to avoid them. This is done easily enough with many contained allergens, such as foods, feathers, and animal dander.

Controlling asthma is much more difficult if the triggers are environmentally produced, like dust and ragweed. In such cases, asthmatics must do their best to minimize exposure by getting rid of dust collectors such as scatter rugs and venetian blinds. Allergic reactions such as hay fever are also sometimes corrected by a series of desensitizing injections, in which gradually increasing amounts of an allergen are introduced to reduce your sensitivity to it. If an allergen is in your work environment, you may have to change jobs or adjust your schedule to avoid the irritant. Moving to another climate is not recommended in most cases, since asthma can occur anywhere.

Exercise-induced asthma (EIA) can result in susceptible individuals after exertion. In the past, physicians told patients with EIA to avoid exercise altogether. Recent research has shown, however, that asthmatics can safely tolerate increases in activity with medication, yet with a decrease in the severity of their attacks.

You can often minimize the effects of EIA by exercising in warm, humid environments, and warming up adequately. Many asthmatics can swim without symptoms; walking and cycling are less likely to cause attacks than running. If continuous exercise precipitates attacks, try stop-start sports such as tennis. Others can reduce the severity of their attacks by breathing slowly through their noses, thus preventing hyperventilation, which is often linked with the onset of EIA. In addition, researchers have noted that certain foods are associated with the onset of EIA. Shellfish,

Exercises to Help You Breathe

At the onset of an asthma attack, you can supplement your asthma medication and try to reduce the severity of the attack with breathing exercises.

RELAXATION BREATHING

Sit in a chair with your back straight and arms propped on your knees so that your upper body is supported and your shoulders Can drop. With your lips puckered, slowly inhale through your nose and exhale through your mouth.

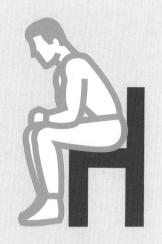

DIAPHRAGMATIC BREATHING

Sit in a chair with one hand held lightly against your stomach. As you inhale, inflate your stomach and feel it push against your hand. As you exhale, deflate your stomach and feel the pressure recede from your hand.

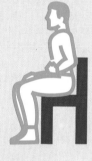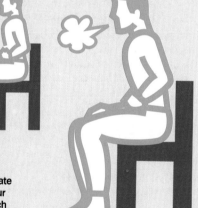

When properly managed, asthma need not hold you back from sports and exercise. In the 1984 Olympics, 67 American athletes — over 10 percent of the total U.S. team — suffered from exercise-induced asthma. Yet this group earned 41 medals. In addition, the U.S. gold medal winner in the 1988 women's heptathlon — a competition that requires endurance, strength and speed in seven track and field events — also had exercise-induced asthma.

celery and peanuts, eaten before exercising, have been most often linked to asthma attacks. Aspirin, too, should be avoided.

Drugs are frequently required to prevent attacks as well as reduce their severity. Bronchodilators, which can be taken orally, inhaled or injected, are used to prevent or mediate attacks by increasing the diameter of air passages and easing the exchange of air in your lungs. Some may require an inhalant called cromolyn, which desensitizes you to allergens.

Asthmatics also report improvements from reducing stress and practicing relaxation techniques, such as those shown on pages 122-123. By lessening anxiety, these techniques help reduce the severity of attacks. You may benefit from performing the exercises shown above.

Back Pain

Your back is a complex composition of bones, cartilage, ligaments, muscles and nerves. Twenty-four separate vertebrae, plus the triangular sacrum located between the hipbones and the nine or ten fused vertebrae of the tailbone, or coccyx, form a flexible, S-shaped curve extending from the base of your skull to your pelvis.

The vertebrae are aligned by ligaments that are supported by muscles. Indeed, much support for your lower back actually comes from your abdominals. Sandwiched between the vertebrae are shock-absorbing, gel-filled discs. The spine serves as a protective conduit for your spinal cord.

Your back is involved in almost every movement you make. It is not surprising that back pain is almost as prevalent as the common cold, affecting 80 percent of all Americans at some time. However, while there are more than 100 known causes of back pain, the majority are rooted in muscle weakness or imbalance. According to one large study, 83 percent of backaches are muscular in origin. Disc problems account for only five to 10 percent of back trouble.

Most backaches begin suddenly, when a simple movement causes an involuntary muscle contraction, or spasm. While excruciating, it causes inflammation that actually serves a protective purpose by immobilizing your back and preventing further damage. Repeated patterns of misuse stemming from inactivity, poor posture habits and improper movements lead to back trouble. Weak abdominal muscles can also predispose you to back pain.

Fortunately, by countering misuse and muscle weakness, you can spare yourself from back pain — or prevent it from recurring. The most important step is exercising to keep the supporting musculature of your back fit and strong. Exercise also helps supply vital nutrients to your discs, delaying age-related deterioration. The exercises in the box at right are specifically designed to strengthen your back-supporting muscles.

Keeping your weight down will lessen the strain on your lower back, since excess weight can overstretch the back-supporting abdominal muscles and ligaments. Improving your posture will reduce the strain on your spine and help correct muscular imbalances. Reducing your stress level will also help, since studies correlate stress with risk of back pain.

Most minor aches are just warnings; reduce strenuous physical activity until they abate, then you should try to incorporate a gradual back-strengthening program. More severe pain usually requires bed rest to allow inflammation to subside; research has found that reclining reduces the pressure on your discs by 70 percent. Aspirin or another analgesic will also reduce inflammation. However, bed rest should be minimized. A recent study found that two days in bed are usually sufficient for most backaches. Longer periods will weaken your muscles, which can lead to more injuries.

Although most cases of back pain do not require medical help, a small percentage of backaches are related to some underlying disease or structural problem. Contact your physician if you experience radiating pain, numbness or tingling in an arm or leg; pain that continues when you lie down; pain that does not improve after two days of bed rest; pain resulting from an accident; pain with vomiting or fever; or backache in a child or elderly person. Performing the exercises shown will give you protection against back pain.

Exercises for a Pain-Free Back

LOWER BACK STRETCH

To stretch your back muscles, lie on your back. Bend your knees and place your feet flat on the floor. Grasp your left knee with both hands and pull it toward your chest. Hold this position for 15-30 seconds. Lower, pause and repeat twice for each leg.

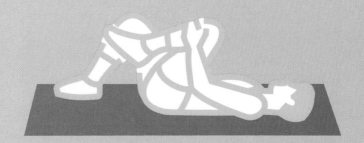

PELVIC TILT

To reduce excess curvature of your back, lie on your back with your feet flat on the floor and knees bent. Flatten the small of your back against the floor by tightening your buttocks and stomach muscles. Hold this position for 5-10 seconds, then relax. Repeat 5 times.

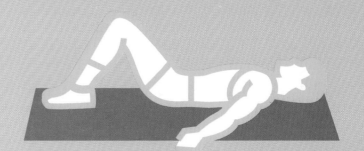

ABDOMINAL CRUNCH

To strengthen your abdominals, lie on your back with your feet flat on the floor, knees bent and arms at your sides. Bend your elbows and place your fingertips against your temples. Raise your shoulder blades off the floor. Return to the starting position. Perform three sets of 10 reps. Work up to three sets of 20 reps.

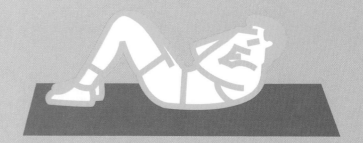

BACK STRENGTHENER

To develop your back extensors, lie on the floor face down with your arms at your sides. Lift your head and chest off the floor; hold this position for five seconds. Rest and repeat. As you gain strength, gradually increase holding time to 10 seconds.

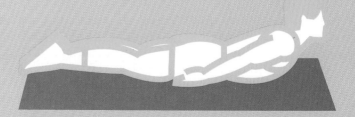

Birth Control

Choosing your method of contraception is a highly personal decision that depends on a number of sometimes conflicting factors. Most people feel that three requirements are of primary concern in birth control: effectiveness, sexual spontaneity and health risks. In general, those methods that are highly effective and allow for the most spontaneity — the contraceptive pill and the intrauterine device (IUD) — also pose the greatest health risks.

A contraceptive's theoretical effectiveness is an estimate of how many pregnancies occur per 100 women using it properly for one year. Actual failure rates may be much higher. For example, the theoretical effectiveness of the diaphragm is 98 percent when fitted and used correctly. However, failure rates in studies that account for misuse result in actual effectiveness as low as 75 percent.

Short of abstaining from sexual intercourse, the surest and safest way to avoid unwanted pregnancies is sterilization. Currently the most common choice of birth control in the United States, sterilization — a vasectomy for men or tubal ligation for women — is relied on by 36 percent of all couples.

Following sterilization, birth-control pills and IUDs are the most effective forms of contraception, yet they can present the most serious side effects. Three independent studies have documented that prolonged use of oral contraceptives led to an increased breast cancer risk. Prior research disputes these findings, and some experts claim that the recent studies are flawed. The pill reduces the chance that a woman will develop ovarian cancer by 10 to 60 percent, and also lessens her risk of developing uterus cancer by approximately 20 to 60 percent.

IUDs have been linked in studies with an increased risk of pelvic inflammatory disease (PID). Not only can PID cause internal scarring that can lead to infertility, it can also be fatal in some cases.

Somewhat less effective and allowing for less sexual spontaneity are the diaphragm, vaginal sponge and condom. However, these methods present almost no health risks, and their failure rates are more often due to improper use rather than cases of product malfunctions.

When choosing a contraceptive, you may want to consider protection from sexually transmitted diseases (STDs), such as genital herpes and acquired immune deficiency syndrome (AIDS). Condoms provide maximum protection against STDs, although the contraceptive jelly or cream used with diaphragms also provides protection. Probably because of this, condom use is on the rise. However, while 60 percent of women report a favorable attitude about them, only 16 percent rely on condom use by their partners for contraception. Condoms may be less popular among men because they must be put on prior to intercourse, and because the latex or lamb cecum material diminishes sensation.

Because your individual health has a large bearing on the optimal contraceptive for you, it is recommended that you make your decision in conjunction with your physician. Fortunately, except for sterilization, these choices are reversible, and many of them can be altered to accommodate your lifestyle.

Methods of Contraception

TYPE	ADVANTAGES	DISADVANTAGES
Birth control pill 98 percent effective, combination pill with synthetic progesterone and estrogen; 90-97 percent effective, mini-pill with synthetic progesterone	• Reduces or eliminates menstrual cramps • Menstrual periods are often light and short • Diminishes risk of fibrocystic breast disease • Combination pill protects against uterine cancer	• Only available by prescription, must be taken on a regular daily schedule • Possibly linked with strokes, blood clots, heart attacks and migraine headaches; smokers and women over 35 are at particularly high risk • May be associated with benign liver tumors and gall bladder disease • May increase the risk of breast cancer for women under 45 • May increase risk of ectopic pregnancy • May produce nausea, fluid retention and breast tenderness during first use • May be associated with diminished sexual response
Cervical cap 96 percent effective when used correctly; otherwise, 75 percent effective	• Can be inserted hours, even a day or two, before intercourse and left in place for up to two days afterward • Small and unobtrusive	• Can be difficult to insert • Must be in place six to eight hours, not over 48 hours after intercourse • Though widely available in Europe, may be difficult to find in the U.S. • Can cause an unpleasant odor
Condom nearly 100 percent effective when partner uses spermicide; 85 percent effective when partner fails to use spermicide	• Protects against sexually transmitted diseases (STDs), including AIDS • Guards against cervical cancer • Available without a prescription	• Can slip off or tear during intercourse • Can diminish sexual sensation
Diaphragm 96 percent effective when fitted and used correctly; otherwise, 75 percent effective	• Very safe • Protects against some STDs • May protect against cervical cancer • Can be inserted up to six hours before intercourse	• Must be fitted by a health professional, only available by prescription • Must be in place for six to eight hours, not over 24 hours after intercourse • Spermicidal cream or jelly must be inserted with an applicator before re-engaging in intercourse when diaphragm is already in place • Increases risk of urinary-tract infection • Must be checked for tiny holes, especially around the rim • Must be refitted after a significant change in weight or pregnancy • Must be cleaned and stored carefully and replaced every few years
Intrauterine device (IUD) 95 percent effective	• Very effective	• Must be fitted and inserted by a doctor, may perforate the uterine wall • Increases risk of pelvic inflammatory disease, which can be life threatening and impair fertility • Increases risk of ectopic pregnancy and miscarriage if pregnancy occurs • May cause cramping and heavy bleeding during menstruation
Spermicidal jelly, cream, foam, suppository 75-90 percent effective alone; almost 100 percent effective with a condom or diaphragm	• Available without prescription • Protects against some STDs	• Must be inserted just before intercourse and reapplied each time before re-engaging • Can cause irritation • Douching or bathing not permitted for six to eight hours after intercourse
Tubal ligation nearly 100 percent effective	• Very effective and safe • Inexpensive, over a long time period	• Often not reversible • Anesthetic used in surgery can present risk of heart attack, cardiac irregularity, internal bleeding and infection • Laparoscopic techniques may cause skin or internal burns, perforation of the uterus, punctured intestine and carbon dioxide embolism • May cause increased menstrual pain and heavy bleeding, necessitating dilation and curettage or a hysterectomy
Vaginal sponge 75-90 percent effective when used correctly	• Spermicide is self-contained • Available without prescription • Can be inserted several hours before intercourse • Protects against some STDs	• Above-average failure rate for women who have given birth • May increase risk of toxic shock syndrome, particularly during menstruation • Can irritate the vaginal lining • Must be left in place for at least six hours, not over 24 hours after intercourse • Can only be used once, may be difficult to remove • Long-term safety studies have not been conducted
Vasectomy nearly 100 percent effective	• Very effective and safe • Inexpensive, over a long time period	• Often not reversible • Additional form of contraception should be used for two months following a vasectomy, or until two negative sperm counts are made

Cholesterol

When the cholesterol levels of 84 long-distance runners were compared to 246 sedentary individuals, it was found that the runners had slightly lower total cholesterol levels. However, the runners' HDL levels, the "good" cholesterol, averaged about 20 mg/dl higher. Similar results have been noted for endurance cyclists, cross-country skiers, ice skaters, swimmers and tennis players. Weight lifting, gymnastics and sprinting, however, do not improve cholesterol levels.

Although it has been implicated as a leading cause of coronary artery disease, cholesterol is not inherently harmful. Indeed, we could not survive without it. A white, odorless, powdery substance that is chemically similar to alcohol, cholesterol is a vital component of cell walls and helps in the production of bile acids and hormones. However, since your liver manufactures all the cholesterol you need — about 1,000 milligrams a day — you do not have to consume it.

Unfortunately, many Americans consume about 400 to 500 milligrams of cholesterol every day, which raises the total amount of cholesterol in their blood. And too much serum cholesterol can be fatal. Scientists at the National Heart, Lung, and Blood Institute say that blood cholesterol levels above 200 to 230 milligrams per deciliter (mg/dl) are associated with increased risk of developing coronary artery disease. One-half of the adults in America have levels above this danger area.

The American Heart Association estimates that the death rate from heart disease declined almost 28 percent between 1976 and 1986. This is thought to be largely the result of reduced levels of smoking and of high-fat foods in the diet and improved control of hypertension. Now, just as millions have reduced their risk of fatal heart attack and stroke by controlling these factors, millions more can benefit from lowering their cholesterol levels.

The first step to control your cholesterol is to get a blood lipid profile, which involves a simple test. Everyone should be tested every three years, beginning at least by age 35. High-risk individuals, such as those with a parent being treated for high cholesterol or those with heart disease in the family, should be tested during childhood or adolescence. Teenagers with high cholesterol should be identified and given dietary intervention.

If you have a high level of cholesterol in your blood, it is to your advantage to lower it. According to a study of nearly 4,000 men aged 35 to 59, lowering overall cholesterol levels by 8.5 percent resulted in a 19 percent lower incidence of heart attack. In other words, for every one percent reduction in your cholesterol, you lower your chance of acquiring heart disease by two percent.

Cholesterol circulates through your bloodstream as water-soluble lipoproteins, which include packages of protein and triglycerides (fats). There are three major classes of lipoproteins. The first, very-low-density lipoprotein (VLDL), is manufactured in your liver and is rich in triglycerides. VLDL carries triglycerides to muscle and fat cells for energy or storage.

Once the triglycerides have been delivered, VLDL becomes low-density-lipoprotein (LDL), the second class of lipoprotein. One particle of LDL contains a single protein molecule, 800 molecules of phospholipids and 500 cholesterol molecules. LDL carries cholesterol through your system, depositing it where it is needed for cell building, and leaving a residue of cholesterol on the arterial walls.

Your liver makes a third type called high-density lipoprotein (HDL), which is a dense package of protein containing less cholesterol than LDL. HDL circulates through your bloodstream and has the beneficial

Lowering Your Cholesterol

Cut down on cholesterol-laden foods, which are always animal products. It is estimated that for every 250 milligrams of cholesterol a person consumes a day, his cholesterol level rises an average 10 mg/dl. Eat lean meats, cut the skin off chicken, and reduce the amount of organ meats and eggs in your diet. One egg yolk contains about 275 milligrams of cholesterol. Remember that some baked or mixed goods may contain eggs, such as pound cake, bran muffins or pancakes. Even though you may avoid butter-fried cheese omelets, you can still be eating eggs and not know it.

◆ Avoid saturated fats as much as possible. These are the fats that are solid at room temperature, such as butter, lard and suet. Fatty meats, whole-milk dairy products, desserts made with shortening and fried foods and creamy soups contain saturated fats, which are also prevalent in coconut, palm and palm kernel oils. Use unsaturated fats such as olive, corn, safflower and sesame oils. (See pages 80-81.)

◆ Eat deep-water ocean fish such as anchovies, herring, salmon, mackerel, sardines, fresh tuna and whitefish. These fish contain omega-3 fatty acids, which some research indicates can help raise your HDL level.

◆ Eat foods high in soluble fiber such as grains, fruits with skins, legumes and vegetables. Foods high in fiber can help raise the HDL level in your blood. (See pages 82-83.)

◆ Exercise regularly. Aerobic exercise such as running, brisk walking, swimming or cycling can raise your level of protective HDL cholesterol while lowering your LDL cholesterol. Exercise can also help you lose weight, which also has a cholesterol-lowering effect. (See pages 84-85.)

◆ Do not smoke. Smoking can increase your total cholesterol and decrease HDL. In addition to its effect on cholesterol levels, smoking is a major independent risk factor in heart disease.

capacity of bringing cholesterol back to your liver for reprocessing or excretion. In other words, LDL carries cholesterol into your system, while HDL removes it.

LDL cholesterol (sometimes referred to as "bad" cholesterol), represents about 60 to 70 percent of your total cholesterol level. HDL cholesterol (the "good" cholesterol), is associated with reduced risk of heart disease; it usually represents 20 to 30 percent of the total. VLDL includes 10 to 15 percent. Because LDL cholesterol is the most abundant in your blood, high total cholesterol is usually associated with a high level of LDL.

Many doctors now believe that your ratio of total cholesterol to HDL is important for assessing your heart disease risk, and that even a low total cholesterol level can result in atherosclerosis if your HDL component is too low. This ratio is determined by dividing the total value by the HDL value. Men should strive for a ratio of 4.5 or less; women should have a ratio less than 3.0.

In some people, high blood cholesterol — hypercholesterolemia — is due to genetic factors and can only be lowered with drug therapy. However, most people with moderately high cholesterol levels can control them through diet and exercise. High serum cholesterol levels are often associated with three dietary factors all too common in the United States: Eating too much saturated fat and dietary cholesterol and being overweight. Eat a diet low in fats, moderate in proteins and high in complex carbohydrates.

Common Colds

Does vitamin C fight the common cold? In one study, researchers gave 190 volunteers capsules containing either a placebo or vitamin C. Some of the subjects knew exactly what they were taking; however, more subjects thought they were receiving vitamin C, yet were not, and the remainder thought they were getting a placebo but were taking vitamin C. The subjects kept track of the colds they suffered. At the end of the study, those who thought they were getting vitamin C — whether or not they actually did — had fewer colds than those who thought they were taking a placebo.

Colds are rarely serious, but they annoy nearly everyone occasionally. The "common cold" is a misleading description for an array of viral infections, most of which cause similar symptoms. These include a sore or scratchy throat, hoarseness, coughing, burning eyes, sneezing, a runny nose and congestion, general malaise, and occasional fever and muscle aches and pains. Inflamed mucous membranes in your nose and throat may cause discomfort, making normal routines and sleep difficult or impossible to accomplish.

At least 200 different cold viruses have been identified by medical science, the most common type being the rhinoviruses. While other cold viruses are more likely to cause winter and early spring colds, rhinoviruses tend to be active in the late summer and early autumn.

You can only catch a rhinovirus from another human. It is not known what makes some people more susceptible to colds than others. Newborns are thought to be immune to about 20 percent of rhinoviruses from their mothers' antibodies, but they soon lose their immunity. Small children are the most susceptible to colds, often having up to eight colds a year of varying durations.

A cold-virus particle is pure RNA — ribonucleic acid — encased in a protein coating. On the protein sheath are molecular receptors that attach to and enter the epithelial cells in the lining of your nose or throat. Once the virus particle has entered the host cell, the RNA imposes its own genetic code on it, turning it into a virus factory. Within eight to 12 hours, the virus particles rupture the cell lining, killing it. The particles then move on to infect neighboring cells.

Your body responds to cold-virus invasions quickly, producing antibodies that attack it. Other substances, such as interferon and histamine, slow the advance of the virus. Most cold symptoms are caused by your immune system's response, not by the virus itself. The incubation period of many colds is one to three days; the illness usually runs its course in about nine days.

Since there are so many different viruses that cause colds, no single vaccine could be effective against all of them. However, people acquire immunity to each particular virus that infects them, so that eventually they become immune to a larger number of cold viruses. By age 60, most people suffer from only one cold a year.

To date, there is no method to prevent or cure colds, but recent breakthroughs in immunology have raised hopes for a cure. Scientists have reported cloning the molecular receptor that rhinoviruses use to infect nasal-passage membranes. This has led to speculation that a nasal spray may be developed that could block the binding cites and prevent infection. Unfortunately, since your nose clears within 15 minutes, the spray may be effective for only a short time. Also, it would not prevent infection by any one of seven other types of cold viruses, which use other receptor cites. Alas, the cure for the common cold is still elusive.

Many commonly held beliefs about colds are false. Getting chilled, for instance, or undergoing rapid weather changes will not bring on a cold — unless you have already been exposed to a virus. In one study, a

Preventing and Treating Colds

◆ Wash your hands frequently if you have a cold or if any member of your family has one. Do not share objects such as drinking glasses, towels or bars of soap with cold sufferers.

◆ Do not take penicillin or other antibiotics to prevent or treat a cold. Antibiotics are effective mainly against bacterial infections, such as strep throat; they can do nothing for a cold, which is a viral infection. A recent survey found that 63 percent of Americans think erroneously that antibiotics kill viruses as well as bacteria. Also, do not take aspirin: It will reduce headache and fever but it will increase your infectiousness.

◆ If you have a cold, make sure that you get an adequate amount of sleep, and rest as much as possible. Refrain from strenuous exercise or sports; physical exhaustion lowers your body's defenses. Also, emotional distress can increase the severity of your symptoms.

◆ If your nose becomes sore from wiping it, apply a petroleum-jelly ointment. Hot soups and other liquids can help loosen nasal mucus and clear congestion.

◆ Do not "starve" a cold or a fever. Maintain your usual diet and drink plenty of fluids. You may take vitamin C supplements if you wish, although a healthy, balanced diet should provide you with adequate nutrients.

group of volunteers was exposed to cold viruses in 40-degree temperatures, while another group was exposed to the same viruses in an 86-degree environment. Both groups caught colds at about the same rate of frequency.

The myth that chilly and rainy weather causes colds probably resulted from the fact that colds seem more prevalent in the fall and winter months. A possible reason for the frequency of colds during these times may be that you spend more time in close contact with others so that viruses have more opportunity to travel from one person to another. School is also in session, and children infect each other and bring colds home to their families.

For decades, scientists believed that cold viruses were spread by droplets in the air by the sneezing and coughing of a cold sufferer. However, researchers have found that colds are more likely to be spread by actual physical contact.

Cold viruses cannot penetrate your skin, nor can they survive on the mucous membranes of your mouth. The only way for a virus to survive and multiply is for it to enter your nose.

How do viruses find your nose? A study showed that up to 90 percent of all cold sufferers had some viruses on their hands. Shaking or holding hands with a cold-infected person is probably the most common method of transmission of the virus, which can survive up to three hours outside your nose. If the healthy person puts his hands to his nose, or rubs his eyes, the virus can pass through his tear duct to his nose.

Because of their close physical contact with one another, family members are the most likely to spread the virus among themselves. If one member of your family has a cold, you have a 25 to 40 percent chance of catching it. Although office workers may have colds at about the same time, tests show that they are usually infected by different viruses.

Dental Care

Optimal dental care requires your daily participation combined with regular checkups. With ongoing oral hygiene, your teeth should last a lifetime; unfortunately, many people neglect dental care until they have pain or symptoms of disease. More than half of all Americans over 60 have no teeth. Unfortunately, according to American Dental Association estimates, fewer than one-third of all Americans brush their teeth more than once a day, and less than half see dentists at least once a year.

The self-care essentials of good oral hygiene are brushing your teeth after eating and flossing daily. Both of these procedures are aimed at preventing plaque buildup — a gummy film comprised of saliva and bacteria that adheres to your teeth and along your gum line. Plaque control is the best way to avoid tooth decay, periodontal disease, gingivitis and bad breath. Within 24 to 36 hours, dental plaque converts to tartar — a hard crust that firmly fixes bacteria to your teeth and irritates your gums.

Tooth decay occurs when the bacteria in plaque break down food particles trapped between teeth, producing an acid that can destroy tooth enamel, causing cavities. Sugar consumption exacerbates this decay process, since the bacteria use it to produce the decay-causing acid. Frequent sugary snacks — especially sticky ones like pastries, cookies, caramels and dried fruits — are greater offenders than sugar consumed with meals. Surprisingly, though, you can treat yourself to an occasional chocolate bar, since it has been found to have some decay-inhibiting properties.

A similar process is at the root of periodontal disease, which is caused by plaque bacteria invading the space between your teeth and gums. In its early stages, this causes gingivitis — red, swollen or bleeding gums. If you have these symptoms, you should see your dentist. Without proper treatment and improved oral hygiene, the impacted bacteria burrow deeper into your gums, ultimately destroying the bone that supports the teeth. As the condition worsens, your teeth loosen and fall out eventually.

Fortunately, the public-health measure of water fluoridation has dramatically reduced dental decay in many Americans: Studies have found that 60 percent of tooth decay can be prevented by children drinking fluoridated water during the first eight years of their lives. Fluoride is an essential micronutrient that protects your teeth by forming decay-resistant mineral crystals in tooth enamel. If the water supply in your community is not fluoridated, your children can benefit from supplementary fluoride tablets included in their diet.

Regardless of your fluoride intake, you must brush your teeth regularly to remove the surface plaque before it turns into tartar. Brush the surfaces of all teeth with short, gentle strokes, with the bristles placed at a 45-degree angle to your teeth. How effectively you use your toothbrush matters more than which kind you use; however, research has found that your teeth and gums will be healthier if you use a small brush that can reach every part of your mouth. Choose soft, round-ended, nylon bristles, and replace your toothbrush every three to four months, since the

Flossing Teeth

While only about one third of adults are reported to floss their teeth on a regular basis, it is an important adjunct to regular brushing. Flossing helps to remove food particles caught between teeth as well as the plaque that builds up on them and along the gum line. When flossing, use about 18 inches of unwaxed dental floss. Wrap most of it around your middle finger of one hand, and wind the remainder around your other middle finger. As you floss, unwind it from the wrapped finger, winding the used floss around the other.

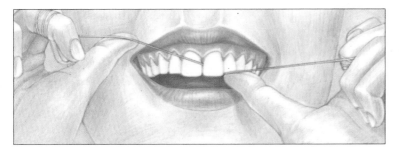

With a gentle, sawing motion, insert the floss between two teeth. Move it slightly below the gum line. Curve the floss around the back of one tooth (*above*). Slide it into the space between your gum and tooth and pull it slightly until you feel resistance. Gently move the floss up and down (*right*). Then curve the floss around the neighboring tooth. Repeat the procedure and slide it out. Continue with the next pair of teeth, flossing until all teeth are clean. Rinse your mouth carefully.

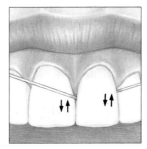

bristles wear out quickly and bend out of shape.

Toothpaste serves as an abrasive that aids in the removal of plaque, food particles and stains. The key element to look for in a toothpaste is type of fluoride compound. Even if your drinking water is fluoridated, daily use of a fluoride toothpaste can help further reduce the incidence of tooth decay.

Many toothpastes marketed as plaque removers are no more effective than regular varieties; only those containing soluble pyrophosphates, which have been shown to inhibit the formation of dental bacteria and tartar, have been approved by the American Dental Association Council of Dental Therapeutics.

Daily flossing of your teeth is also crucial for plaque removal and maintaining healthy gums. Flossing removes the hard-to-reach food particles and plaque that forms between your teeth and just below your gum line — where periodontal disease starts. See the box (*above*) for directions on how to floss properly.

Because of the prevalence of "dentist phobia," many people do not visit their dentists on a regular basis, which allows trouble to mount and fulfills their fears that dental treatments will be necessary. No matter how diligent your oral hygiene, biannual visits to your dentist for a full examination and professional cleaning are essential elements of preventive dental care.

Doctors

To ensure that you stay healthy, you need to have ready access to all that modern medicine has to offer. The best way is to find the right primary-care physician — the doctor who will meet your general health-care needs and act as intermediary to the complete medical community.

A primary-care physician should be competent in handling most medical problems that you encounter, know your medical history and keep your records on file. Most are either internists or family practitioners, but you might also be able to find a general practitioner — the kind of doctor who does not specialize — although they are becoming less available.

Family practitioners are specialists who handle a wide range of problems, treating most acute and chronic illnesses, broken bones and even offering psychological counseling for such conditions as alcoholism. In addition, many family practitioners provide obstetrical care, and all treat children as patients. Internists specialize in adult medical problems; they have more advanced training in diagnosis than family practitioners. And they may further specialize in heart disease, diabetes, cancer or arthritis, for example.

Someone who is licensed to practice medicine may be either a medical doctor (M.D.), or an osteopath (D.O.), who is trained similar to a medical doctor, and can be certified by regular medical-specialty boards. Osteopaths have been gaining wider acceptance and availability within the medical community.

Your primary-care physician should be a good resource in the event that you need a specialist. He should be able to function as a coordinator with a number of different doctors. However, using a specialist for basic medical care is expensive. And relying on emergency-room doctors will provide you with less-than-ideal care, since they will not have access to your medical records. They are trained to handle emergencies, not general medical problems.

Begin by making a list of doctors by asking your friends about theirs, keeping in mind that your friends' needs may be quite different from yours. More reliable sources include other physicians, nurses or health-care professionals. Referrals by other medical professionals indicate that a physician has a good reputation among his or her colleagues. You can also call medical societies and hospitals for referrals.

Once you have a list of physicians, you must make an essential judgment of each one's technical abilities. There are three areas to consider: Where he or she has staff privileges, if he is board certified and his training. (All physicians should be board certified, which means that they have passed qualifying examinations.) This information is available either in the *AMA Directory of Physicians* or the Marquis *Directory of Medical Specialists*.

In some areas, a physician may be a "fellow," which means that he or she has undertaken some advanced training, as indicated by initials such as "FACP" (Fellow of the American College of Physicians). The initials "PC" stand for professional corporation and do not reflect a qualifying degree or affiliation.

If a physician has staff privileges at a university hospital, it is likely that he will have teaching and research

Choosing a Specialist

Your primary-care physician, a doctor with a wide clinical background and who knows your medical history, is equipped to attend to most of your medical needs. While your family doctor may have substantial knowledge in many branches of medicine and specific understanding of you as a patient, he may sometimes refer you to a specialist who is more deeply experienced in a specific area of medicine. The following is a list of some common specialists:

- **Allergist.** An expert who is concerned with the diagnosis and treatment of allergies.

- **Cardiologist.** A physician who specializes in diseases and disorders of the heart and blood vessels.

- **Dermatologist.** A specialist who diagnoses and treats diseases and disorders of the skin.

- **Endocrinologist.** An expert in problems with the hormonal system, growth and development.

- **Gastroenterologist.** One who treats diseases and disorders of the digestive system.

- **Neurologist.** A doctor who specializes in diseases and disorders of the nervous system.

- **Obstetrician-Gynecologist.** A physician who is concerned with human reproduction and the female reproductive system.

- **Oncologist.** A cancer specialist.

- **Orthopedist.** A doctor who treats injuries and diseases of the bones, joints and skeletal system.

- **Otolaryngologist.** An expert in problems with the ears, nose or throat.

- **Psychiatrist.** A physician who diagnoses and treats emotional and mental disorders.

- **Rheumatologist.** A specialist in arthritis and other inflammatory diseases.

- **Urologist.** A physician who treats disorders of the urinary-tract organs and, in men, problems in the reproductive system.

responsibilities. While this is valuable for a specialist, you might not require it for primary care.

You can also find out most of this information by calling a doctor's office. Inquire about fees, office procedures — which tests can be done in the office — other doctors in a group practice, if applicable, and insurance practices. Ask if he accepts Medicare, Medicaid or insurance-policy payments.

Arrange to meet the physician. You can evaluate his accessibility, how easy it is to schedule appointments, how long you may expect to wait and the office environment. Assess the physician's attitude — whether or not he is easy to talk to, if he inspires confidence, and if he is willing to answer your questions. Make sure that another doctor is available when the physician is away. Ask if he makes referrals and suggests second opinions when appropriate. You might also ask if the physician has ever been convicted of malpractice. For additional tips for choosing a doctor or specialist, see the box *(above)*.

Driving Safety

utomobile accidents are the leading cause of accidental deaths. In the United States, an estimated 60 percent of them could be avoided, or their severity reduced, if people drove defensively and always used seat belts. Studies have shown that seat belts could save about 18,000 lives and greatly reduce the more than 1.5 million injuries that occur annually.

Mandatory seat-belt use in many states has saved almost 7,000 lives between 1984 and 1987. A U.S. Government safety regulation requiring that all new automobiles be equipped with passive restraints — either belts that automatically protect the occupant once the door is closed or air bags — will save even more lives. When buying a new car, select one with an air bag. At 35 mph, a crash is

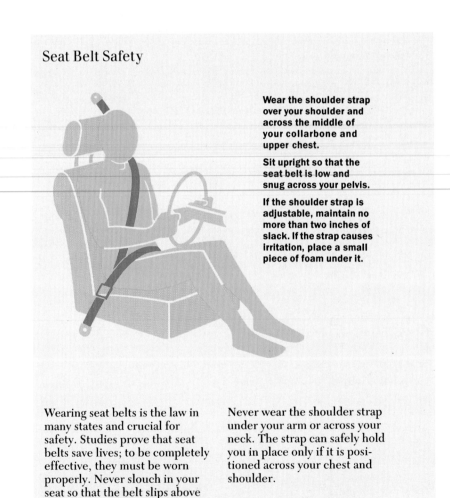

Seat Belt Safety

Wear the shoulder strap over your shoulder and across the middle of your collarbone and upper chest.

Sit upright so that the seat belt is low and snug across your pelvis.

If the shoulder strap is adjustable, maintain no more than two inches of slack. If the strap causes irritation, place a small piece of foam under it.

Wearing seat belts is the law in many states and crucial for safety. Studies prove that seat belts save lives; to be completely effective, they must be worn properly. Never slouch in your seat so that the belt slips above your pelvis. In an accident, your pelvis can withstand the pressure of 20-50 times your body weight.

Never wear the shoulder strap under your arm or across your neck. The strap can safely hold you in place only if it is positioned across your chest and shoulder.

Be sure to buckle up *before* you drive. Do not attempt to buckle your seat belt while driving.

so severe that the head of the driver almost always hits the steering wheel, even if he is securely restrained with a seat belt. Unfortunately, the law does not require manufacturers to install passive restraints in vans, minivans, and sport-utility vehicles; despite the increasing popularity and prevalence of these varieties.

Currently, 76 percent of all Americans still do not buckle up regularly. And even when the automatic belts become available, consumer advocates predict that, because many are so inconvenient, most people will use them manually or not at all — a dangerous practice considering that even if you have excellent driving skills, you still have a one-in-three chance of being in a serious accident.

Some people do not wear seat belts because they believe that they can trap them in a car or prevent them from being thrown clear. In fact, fewer than one in a thousand accidents involve any danger of being trapped in a car that is immersed in water or on fire. During such accidents, wearing a seat belt will give you the greatest chance of remaining conscious and free of injury so that you will be able to take action if it is necessary.

In addition, studies show that persons who are thrown clear are 25 times more likely to be killed or seriously injured as those who are not restrained by seat belts. After all, to be thrown clear usually means being thrown out the door or through the windshield. Also, if you land on the street, you risk being run over by another car. Four out of five people who were killed when they were thrown clear would have lived had they been able to stay in the car. See the illustration *(opposite)* for more information about automobile safety.

Children pose a special safety concern, since motor-vehicle-related fatalities are the leading cause of death and serious injury in children over six months old. Never hold a baby or small child on your lap; even in a 30-mph crash, a 15-pound baby can be propelled forward with a force of 450 pounds. Car seats for children under four years of age are now mandatory in all states.

Probably the best precaution is not to drink alcohol and drive. Even one drink will impair your ability to make quick decisions. And it is a myth that drunk drivers do not get hurt in accidents; they are more likely to be hurt or killed than sober drivers. Unfortunately, you cannot prevent other drivers from drinking. If you suspect that another driver is drunk, stay as far away from his car as possible. If his car is coming toward you, slow down, move to the right and stop; flash your lights and blow your horn to get his attention.

Adjusting your speed for road conditions is a cardinal rule. This will allow you time to avoid making sudden moves, which can cause skids. If you must brake on a slippery road, depress the brake pedal repeatedly and gently. If you skid, take your foot off the accelerator and steer in the direction that the rear of the car is skidding until you regain control.

Many potentially dangerous car malfunctions can be easily averted by regular maintenance. Tune up your engine every 10,000 miles. Change the oil and oil filter every 5,000 miles. Many other problems can be avoided if you inspect the tires, brake and signal lights and head lamps regularly and replace them accordingly.

Eating Disorders

People develop eating disorders when their perceptions about food assume obsessive significance that has little to do with nutrition. In these cases, eating behavior becomes externally motivated — by a desire to be thin, to compensate for a frustrated emotional need or as a response to stress. The common manifestations of such emotionally based eating habits are self-imposed starvation, which is known as anorexia nervosa, and bulimia, or binge eating followed by vomiting and/or using laxatives.

Anorexia and bulimia have reached epidemic proportions among adolescents over the past 15 years. Both are recent disorders affecting young women primarily and occurring almost exclusively in industrial countries. Experts believe that some of the forces behind these aberrant behaviors are cultural, resulting from our modern society's emphasis on the desirability of being as thin as possible, as dictated by fashion.

With such expectations, it is not surprising that women's feelings about their bodies are affected by their weight and shape, and few of them are content with their physical condition. A recent survey of nearly 9,000 women found that 53 percent were dissatisfied with their bodies. For some young women, these same feelings evolve into an obsession that can lead to anorexia or bulimia.

What is Anorexia?

Anorexia nervosa, which now affects more than one of every 100 women, is self-starvation to the point that a woman's weight is at least 15 percent less than the average for her age and height, and sometimes as much as 35 percent less. Most anorexics come from middle- to upper-class families and, prior to their eating disorder, were viewed as both intelligent and well-behaved children.

Anorexics have an intense fear of weight gain, regardless of how underweight they are. Accompanying this delusion is a disturbance in the way the woman perceives her body. Even when emaciated, anorexics will claim to be overweight. Anorexia almost always causes hormonal disturbances; the most common result is amenorrhea, which is the cessation of menstruation. An estimated 20 percent of anorexics die from starvation or complications attributable to their disorder. See the chart (*opposite*) for the warning signs of anorexia.

The Dangers of Bulimia

Unlike anorexics, bulimics usually maintain their approximately normal weight. However, they are equally concerned with their weight and body shape. Bulimic behavior includes bouts of binge eating, or rapid consumption of large amounts of food. To avoid becoming fat, bulimics alternate binges with dangerous purges — bouts of dieting or fasting, obsessive exercising, self-induced vomiting or using laxatives or diuretics, all of which can wreak havoc in your mouth, stomach and bowel.

Bulimia is a more prevalent disorder than anorexia and, while most of its victims are women, bulimia is also more common in men than anorexia. Among college women, the number of bulimics range between 5 and 20 percent.

The families of bulimics often have a history of alcoholism, depression or obesity, and bulimics frequently abuse alcohol or drugs, or they are sexually promiscuous. Almost 90 percent of bulimics exhibit symptoms of depression, such as an inability to enjoy physical or intellectual pursuits, seem withdrawn, complain of ill health and fail to plan ahead for anything.

Treating Eating Disorders

Both anorexics and bulimics require nutritional counseling combined with psychotherapy to delve into the underlying issues of their diminished self-esteem, low sense of personal control, depression and deluded perceptions about their bodies. Family therapy can be especially useful in the treatment of anorexia, since the disease is often a manifestation of family problems. Behavior therapy has also proven effective for both forms of eating disorders.

Medical intervention — particularly in cases of anorexia — is sometimes necessary. Depending on the degree of emaciation, dehydration or electrolyte imbalance, different treatments can be effective, ranging from antidepressive drug therapies to hospitalization in extreme cases.

Drastic measures can be averted if symptoms are recognized early and appropriate counseling is undertaken, but both anorexia and bulimia can be difficult to diagnose in their early stages. Unusual weight loss, peculiar eating habits, dieting in young women or menstrual irregularities for over three months should be brought to the attention of a doctor.

Warning Signs of Anorexia and Bulimia

ANOREXIA NERVOSA

FOOD RELATED

- Self-imposed starvation to achieve self-control; caloric intake often less than 100 calories per day
- Often skips meals
- Preoccupation with food and calorie counting
- Denies hunger and fatigue
- Excessive exercise to avoid weight gain
- Considers only certain foods (often low-calorie vegetables and lean meats) as acceptable to eat; eats strictly limited portions of food
- Avoids carbohydrates and fats
- Exhibits unusual behavior such as cutting food into extremely small pieces, lingering over small meals for long periods of time and hoarding food

PHYSICAL HEALTH

- Weight about 85 percent or less than desirable
- Menstruation ceases for three or more consecutive months
- Cold intolerance
- Nausea, constipation
- Dehydration, dry skin, thin, brittle, dry hair
- Low blood pressure
- Heart becomes weaker, heartbeat may become irregular
- Edema (fluid in body tissue that produces swelling)
- Muscles deteriorate
- Mental dullness and apathy
- Possible impairment of sexual performance and sex drive
- Impaired nutrient absorption—diarrhea may occur when normal eating is resumed
- Electrolyte imbalance
- Digestive-track lining atrophies
- Sleep disturbances
- Immune dysfunction

BULIMIA NERVOSA

FOOD RELATED

- Binge-eating episodes at least twice per week for three months or longer, usually in private
- Frequent self-induced vomiting
- Binges usually follow strict dieting or fasting bouts
- Feeling out of control of eating behavior
- Guilt and depression
- Skips meals
- Foods chosen for binging are high in sugar and fat
- Overconcern with ideal body weight
- Uses diuretics or laxatives after binges
- Binging to deal with stress
- Preoccupation with food
- Frequent alcohol use
- Discomfort when eating with others

PHYSICAL HEALTH

- Erosion of tooth enamel from stomach acid
- Frequent weight fluctuations (usually more than 10 pounds from binge-and-fast episodes)
- Bloating, swollen feet and hands, fatigue, headache, abdominal pain or nausea following binging
- Vomiting may cause fluid and electrolyte imbalance, leading to kidney problems or abnormal heartbeat
- Kidney failure resulting from kidney and bladder infections
- Stomach or esophagus rupture or tear
- Salivary glands, esophagus or pharynx may become irritated or infected from frequent vomiting
- Lower-intestinal-tract injuries from use of potent laxatives
- Dehydration
- Chronic sore throat and swollen glands
- Irregular menstrual cycle

Eating Out

Increasingly, restaurant fare has become a time-saving and relaxing necessity: It is estimated that most Americans now dine out an average of once a day. Yet, while many people make nutritious meals at home, they often ignore healthy eating habits when dining in restaurants. Even people who would not think of eating deep-fried and heavily salted foods at home may not be aware of all the ingredients or methods of preparation of their meal when they dine in restaurants.

However, dining out need not mean forfeiting a healthy diet: Creative ordering is often the key to maintaining it when away from your own kitchen. For instance, you can order a selection of appetizers and side

Guide to Healthy Dining Out: Meals

	CHOOSE	AVOID
Breakfast	Whole-wheat toast, English muffins, bagels, bran muffins, pancakes or waffles with plain, low-fat yogurt and fresh fruit toppings, hot cereals such as oatmeal, bran flakes or shredded wheat with skim milk; jam, preserves or low-fat cottage cheese on breads	Eggs, butter, cream cheese, bacon, sausage, ham, fast-food biscuits, doughnuts, croissants, Danish pastries, hash browns and granola
Lunch, dinner		
Salads	All types of fresh vegetable or fruit salads, protein-rich beans for main-course salad; for dressing, lemon juice, low-calorie or oil and vinegar; ask for dressing on the side and dilute with vinegar	Potato, macaroni or tuna salads in mayonnaise, marinated vegetables, eggs, cheese, bacon bits, butter-fried croutons, avocado, ready-made pasta salads and meats; creamy salad dressings with mayonnaise or sour cream
Soups	Tomato- or broth-based soups such as minestrone, chicken noodle and vegetable; split pea and lentil soups with crackers or bread make low-fat carbohydrate-rich meals	Cream-based soups such as New England clam chowder; sodium-restricted dieters should avoid soups since most contain large amounts of sodium
Appetizers	Raw vegetables, melon, steamed seafood, popcorn without butter or salt	Cheese and crackers, pâtés, nuts, corn or potato chips
Main courses	Broiled fish and shellfish, skinless white-meat poultry or lean red meat; meatless dishes such as pasta or rice with vegetables or legumes, no cream sauce or butter; food that is baked, steamed, roasted or dry-broiled in lemon juice or wine; ask that fat and skin be removed from meat or poultry before cooking; lean cold cuts include turkey or chicken breast; mustard and vegetable slices instead of mayonnaise or dressing on sandwiches; pita and whole-grain breads and English muffins	Organ meats, duck, goose, poultry with skin and processed meats; food that is fried, creamed, crispy, braised, escalloped, buttery, pan-fried, marinated in oil, basted, in a pot pie, prime, stewed, parmesan or sautéed; food in butter, cheese, gravy, hollandaise, mayonnaise or cream sauces; casseroles and quiches; sodium-restricted dieters should avoid foods that are smoked, pickled, in broth or in a tomato base; fatty cold cuts such as bologna and salami; cheese and dressing or mayonnaise; sandwiches on croissants or biscuits
Side dishes	Steamed, boiled, baked or raw vegetables; low-fat yogurt topping for baked potatoes	Vegetables or starches prepared with fats (oil, butter, mayonnaise or sour cream) or cheese; coleslaw, potato and macaroni salad
Desserts	Fresh fruit, fruit ices, sherbet, angelfood cake; skim or low-fat milk in coffee	Pastries, cakes, pies, cookies; ice cream, custard and cheese made from whole milk

dishes — such as steamed vegetables, rice, salad and a small portion of meat — instead of a full dinner. Also, ask the chef to remove the skin from chicken or broil a fish fillet rather than fry it in butter.

Cafeterias and fast-food places often present the greatest challenges to people who follow the rules of good nutrition. Many cafeterias, for instance, display desserts first and only later offer healthier, more nutritious foods. If possible, preview cafeteria lines to survey the choices or go through the line in reverse.

Now many restaurants have salad bars. But beware: In addition to lettuce and fresh vegetables, they offer cheese, hard-boiled eggs, bacon bits, ham, croutons, mayonnaise, sour cream and oil-based dressings and other items that can turn any healthy meal into a highly caloric and fatty junket. Instead, choose only fresh vegetables and avoid the potato salad, coleslaw and high-fat, high-sodium garnishes. The charts on these two pages can help you make nutritious food choices in virtually any type of restaurant.

Guide to Healthy Dining Out: Restaurants

	CHOOSE	AVOID
Chinese	Stir-fried or steamed chicken, fish, vegetables or bean curd; clear soups with bean curd, vegetables, soft noodles and steamed brown rice; ask that MSG and salt not be added	Deep-fried foods such as egg rolls and noodles; egg foo young and any item with lobster or sweet and sour sauce; sauces or soups with beaten egg; high-fat items such as spare ribs, shrimp toast and Peking duck; Szechwan and Hunan dishes are often deep-fried and high in fat; soy sauce or MSG
Fast food	Salad bars; plain hamburger on a bun with tomato, lettuce and onion without dressing; pizza slice topped with vegetables	Double-decker burgers, cheeseburgers, hot dogs; fried foods including fries, chicken and fish sandwiches; milkshakes; pizza with processed meats
French	Seafood cooked in wine sauce, steamed vegetables, stock-based soups, sorbet and french bread without butter	Pâtés, duck, organ meats; foods cooked in sauces with butter, eggs or cream such as bearnaise or bechamel; French onion soup, quiches and pastries; nouvelle cuisine is usually very high in fat
Italian	Pasta with vegetables, marinara (tomato-based) or red clam sauce, broiled shellfish and veal or chicken in wine- or stock-based sauces; mixed green salads with dressing on the side, Italian bread without butter and fruit ices	Pasta with butter or cream sauce; processed or ground meats; deep-fried mozzarella and zucchini sticks, veal parmesan, osso buco; fettuccine Alfredo, foods topped with mozzarella cheese or deep-fried; garlic bread, cheesecake, cannoli, gelati, zuppa anglaise
Japanese	Tofu (bean curd) dishes, sashimi (raw fish) and sushi (raw fish and rice) without soy sauce; yakimono, which means the food is broiled	Deep-fried foods such as tempura, sodium-rich sauces, including soy sauce, and fish roe
Mexican	Baked corn tortillas, seviche (fish marinated in lime juice and seasoned with spices), gazpacho and salsa	Refried beans and fried flour tortillas made with lard; cheese, avocado or sour cream; deep-fried taco or tostada shells
Steakhouse	Lean London broil, filet mignon or round steak with no butter added and fat trimmed before cooking; baked potato with yogurt	Meat broiled or pan-fried with fat; sirloin steak, prime ribs, lamb chops, gravy, sour cream and french fries

Eye Care

Most people value their eyesight more than any other sense. However, eye care is often a neglected aspect of general health maintenance, leading to many unnecessary cases of vision loss. In fact, protecting your vision is simply a matter of having your eyes examined regularly and practicing safety when performing sports or activities that might endanger your eyesight (see the box at right).

Regular eye exams not only help maintain your visual acuity, they screen for more serious eye conditions that can lead to problems or blindness, most of which can be controlled with early detection and treatment. Also, by examining your eyes, doctors can detect and monitor certain systemic illnesses, such as hypertension, diabetes and even some types of cancer.

Infants' eyes should be examined during routine physicals; preschoolers should have one thorough eye exam between the ages of three and four; thereafter, you should have your eyes checked every 18 months to two years. Healthy adults should have routine exams as outlined on the chart on page 103, and have both a glaucoma and visual acuity test at least every two years after they reach the age of 40.

There are three kinds of eye-care specialists: They are ophthalmologists, optometrists and opticians. An ophthalmologist is a certified doctor of medicine who specializes in the medical and surgical care of eyes. Ophthalmologists not only do vision testing and prescribe corrective lenses, they also diagnose and treat eye disorders ranging from minor infections and inflammations such as conjunctivitis to more serious conditions like glaucoma. Optometrists are not medical doctors, but are required to attend a special four-year school of optometry. They are licensed to perform vision testing and prescribe corrective lenses, and in some states, they can treat minor eye diseases. An optometrist refers you to an ophthalmologist if he or she suspects any serious disorder. Opticians are not trained to do vision testing; they are technicians who fill prescriptions for eyeglasses or contact lenses.

Testing Your Vision

During an eye exam, your visual acuity is compared to the 20/20 standard, which is an established measure of visual sharpness that means you can read a designated line of print when standing 20 feet from an eye chart. If you cannot read the print at 20 feet, you are asked to look at print of progressively larger letters, until they are legible. If, for example, you have 20/100 vision, the smallest print you can read when standing 20 feet from the vision chart could be read by someone with 20/20 vision when standing 100 feet from the chart.

Less than 20/20 vision is almost always due to faulty focusing ability of your eyes — the most common cause of vision impairment. When your eyes focus optimally, your lenses, which are located directly behind your irises, focus images precisely onto your retinas, the layers of light-sensitive cells at the backs of your eyeballs. There are four basic vision abnormalities: nearsightedness, or myopia; farsightedness, or hyperopia; astigmatism; and the very common presbyopia.

Nearsightedness, which causes blurry vision for distances, is the most common focusing disorder; it happens when your lenses focus images in front of your retinas. In farsightedness, the opposite occurs: Images are focused behind your retinas, making it difficult for you to see close objects. Astigmatism is caused by irregular corneal or lens curvatures, which leads to variable blurred vision. In presbyopia, the ability of your eyes to change focus is impaired as a result of lens rigidity and weakened eye muscles. This problem gradually develops with age and will eventually affect almost everyone; one survey found that 97 percent of Americans over 45 need corrective glasses for reading.

Fortunately, all of these focusing problems can easily be corrected. There are many options in corrective lenses, ranging from trifocal eyeglasses to extended-wear contact lenses that can remain in your eyes for up to a month. You should decide which corrective measures are best for you with your eye doctor.

Eye Diseases

While both optometrists and ophthalmologists are qualified to test your visual acuity, only ophthalmologists can perform the medical elements of visual exams that detect eye diseases as well as some systemic illnesses. The eye diseases that are most prevalent are glaucoma, cataracts, amblyopia, or "lazy eye," and conjunctivitis.

Glaucoma is caused by excess pressure in your eyes, which can damage your optic nerves; 12 percent of blindness cases in the United

Protecting Your Eyes from Injury

More than one million people suffer eye injuries each year; tragically, they account for 10 percent of all cases of blindness. However, an estimated 90 percent of these injuries are preventable. The following tips may save your eyesight:

◆ Forty-five percent of all eye injuries occur around the home, involving everyday household products. Always read instructions carefully when using cleaning fluids, ammonia or any other household chemical; point all spray nozzles away from you before using them. Wear protective goggles when handling especially strong chemicals.

◆ Never stand alongside or in front of a moving lawn mower, and be sure to pick up rocks and stones in its path. Steer clear of low-hanging branches.

◆ Never use explosive fireworks or allow children to ignite or play with them. Use caution even when igniting nonexplosive fireworks such as sparklers.

◆ Eye-related sports injuries are increasing; wear protective safety goggles when playing any racquet sport or basketball. In contact sports, wear helmets or face protectors. If you wear contact lenses, use safety goggles during all sports activities. In addition, wear protective goggles in your workshop or when making automotive repairs.

◆ Ultraviolet rays from the sun or sunlamps can damage your retinas and are implicated in causing cataracts. When you are in the sun or use a sunlamp, wear sunglasses that block all ultraviolet light. See pages 124-125 for tips on buying sunglasses.

◆ When purchasing eyeglasses or sunglasses, be sure that they meet FDA regulations for impact-resistant lenses.

States are caused by this disorder. Cataracts cause a gradual clouding of your eye lenses. Eighty percent of Americans who are 65 or older have some noticeable clouding of vision; about half of them have cataracts that reduce their visual acuity to 20/30 or less. Eventually, your lenses may have to be surgically removed to maintain vision; they are replaced by plastic implants, contact lenses or eyeglasses. Cataract surgery is the most common form of surgery for Americans over 65.

Amblyopia is usually a muscular disorder that causes crossed eyes or walleyes in children. If not attended to early, it can damage vision permanently. Finally, any disorder of your conjunctivas — the thin tissues that cover the fronts of your eyes and the insides of your eyelids — is termed conjunctivitis. Pinkeye, the most common form of conjunctivitis, causes unsightly redness, and discharge and uncomfortable itching, but poses no long-term dangers; other forms may be more serious.

Regardless of when you last had your eyes examined, you should see your eye-care practitioner if you find yourself squinting or blinking excessively, stumbling or rubbing your eyes. Also, seek attention if you seem especially sensitive to bright lights or experience blurred or foggy vision, lose peripheral sight or see rainbow-colored halos around lights. Often, signs of peripheral vision loss are evident if you have trouble parallel parking your car and are involved in a series of accidents.

Fats

Technically called lipids, fats are in solid or liquid forms. All are insoluble in water and high in calories. Although carbohydrates supply your main source of food energy, fats are the most concentrated source with nine calories per gram; carbohydrates and proteins have four calories per gram. Your body stockpiles fat as its primary form of stored energy and body insulation, but excess fat swells your adipose cells, causing weight gain. Extra calories from carbohydrates and proteins are also stored as body fat, but since fat contains more calories per gram, you are more likely to eat too many calories if your diet is high in fat.

Contrary to what many Americans believe, however, fat is an essential ingredient in a healthy diet. You need a certain amount of fat to maintain good health, and almost all foods contain at least a small amount of it.

Fats are responsible for carrying the four fat-soluble vitamins: A, E, D and K; they maintain healthy hair and skin; fats regulate your blood cholesterol level; and they delay hunger pangs by slowing the passage of food from the stomach. Moreover, fats supply essential fatty acids, which your body must get from foods, since it cannot make them. Essential fatty acids are also the raw materials for several hormones, including prostaglandins, which help control blood pressure and other vital bodily functions. Linoleic acid is the most important essential fatty acid, since it is necessary for the proper growth and development of infants; adults need it to maintain their skin and liver.

While fat is necessary for good nutrition, diets high in fat have been related to increased risk of cancer, especially of the colon and breast, as well as gall bladder and coronary heart disease and obesity. Those who are overweight are also at a greater risk of developing cancer of the uterus, hypertension, diabetes, stroke and other health problems.

Americans consume more fat than nearly any other people in the world, as much as 37 percent of all calories, mostly from animal products. Our fat intake has increased significantly since the turn of the century, while our consumption of complex carbohydrates, which come from plants, has decreased.

Saturated vs. Unsaturated Fat

Not all fats are alike. A saturated fat is primarily made up of saturated fatty acids, those with the highest number of hydrogen atoms and no "empty spots," or points of unsaturation. Highly saturated fats come primarily from animal sources, including butter, whole milk and meats; coconut and palm vegetable oils are also highly saturated. All of these fats are usually solid when they are at room temperature.

Unsaturated fatty acids vary according to their degree of saturation. They can be monounsaturated, having one point of unsaturation on their fatty acid chains, or polyunsaturated, with two or more points that are unsaturated. Good sources of unsaturated fatty acids are plants and fish. The monounsaturated variety is found in olive, peanut and avocado oils; polyunsaturates can be found in corn, safflower and sesame oils. Unsaturated fats are generally liquid at room temperature and may become rancid quickly.

Heart Disease and Fats

Saturated fats have been most closely implicated in heart disease. They stimulate the production of LDL ("bad") cholesterol and raise overall cholesterol levels. For this reason, even if you avoid cholesterol in your diet, but still consume a lot of saturated fats, your blood cholesterol levels will probably remain high. See pages 64-65 for more detailed information on cholesterol.

Hydrogenation is a manufacturing process that adds hydrogen atoms to unsaturated fats, making them more saturated. The fats in margarines and shortenings are often hydrogenated to make them harder and increase their shelf life. Depending on the degree of hydrogenation, however, these artificially saturated vegetable fats are often just as harmful as animal fats.

Polyunsaturated fats tend to lower the amount of artery-clogging LDL cholesterol in your blood, as well as the beneficial HDL cholesterol, thus reducing the total amount in your body. Moreover, omega-3 polyunsaturated fatty acids found in certain fish and shellfish offer an additional benefit: They make your blood platelets less likely to clot, reducing your chance of an artery blockage and heart attack.

Monounsaturated fats, such as olive oil, may also reduce the amount of bad LDL cholesterol in your blood, according to some recent studies. Whatever degree of saturation, any kind of fat increases your chance of becoming overweight or

Reducing Your Fat Intake

The following tips, which are based on United States Department of Agriculture guidelines, will help you reduce your intake of fat, especially the saturated variety.

◆ Read labels carefully to determine both the amount and type of fats in packaged foods. To determine the number of calories that come from fat, multiply the number of grams per serving by nine. Then divide this number by the total calories per serving to get the percentage of fat calories.

◆ Limit your intake of fats and oils, particularly those high in saturated fat, such as butter, cream, lard, heavily hydrogenated fats (some margarines), shortenings, and foods containing coconut or palm oil. Choose a margarine that has at least twice as much polyunsaturated fat as saturated.

◆ You do not have to alter your diet dramatically to cut down on fat intake. Follow these nutrition pointers for selecting and preparing foods:

- Substitute fish, chicken or turkey breast (without the skin), or dried beans for red meat.
- Select lean meats and trim all visible fat.
- Use skim or low-fat milk and milk products such as cheese.
- Broil, bake or boil instead of frying foods in fat.
- Avoid fat-laden snack foods.

obese, which is a risk factor in cardiovascular disease.

The Cancer Link

The relationship between fat intake and certain types of cancer is more controversial than the link to heart disease. Many scientists have noted that, with a few exceptions, countries where people eat a lot of fat also have the highest cancer rates. American women, for instance, have a six-times-higher rate of breast cancer than Japanese women, who eat much less fat. Indeed, in one study of 41 countries, researchers found almost a direct relationship between the total fat consumed in various societies and the mortality rate from breast cancer. Some studies have suggested that a high-fat diet also increases your risk of colon cancer and possibly the development of cancer of the ovary, uterus and prostate.

Researchers are uncertain why high-fat diets are associated with cancer. Their theories include that fat may affect the secretion of some sex hormones, which may then cause cancer to develop in your reproductive organs. Moreover, high-fat diets increase the amount of cholesterol and bile acids in your colon, which may be converted by bacteria into carcinogenic by-products that promote the growth of cancer cells.

How Much Fat?

The American Heart Association and American Cancer Society say that no more than 30 percent of your total calories should come from fats. Furthermore, the AHA recommends that your fat intake consist of equal amounts of saturated, monounsaturated and polyunsaturated fats. The box *(above)* offers tips to help you eat a healthy level of fat.

Fiber

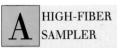
Fiber contributes few if any nutrients to your body and it provides you with virtually no energy, yet it is one of the most beneficial elements of a balanced diet. Fiber is an aid to digestion; it can help you control your weight; and it appears to prevent or alleviate a range of disorders, including heart disease and colon cancer. Consuming fiber is essential for wellness, but most Americans consume far too little of it.

Fiber comes exclusively from plant sources, such as vegetables, nuts, grains, fruits and seeds. The bran in whole-grain breads and cereals is probably the most familiar form of fiber, but, in fact, dietary fiber is a complex assortment of substances that have varied physical and chemical properties. They have one aspect in common: All fiber passes through your system undigested. Unlike other basic nutrients, fiber resists digestive enzymes and so travels through your small and large intestines without being converted into energy. Some fiber is insoluble, traveling through your entire digestive tract unchanged; other soluble types are broken down by bacteria in your large intestine and changed into products your body absorbs.

Researchers have found that these two basic types of fiber produce different effects in your body. Cellulose, one insoluble fiber that is most commonly found in whole grains, acts like a sponge. As it passes through your system, cellulose absorbs many times its weight in water. It is also partially fermented by bacteria in your large intestine. Both actions help produce a large, soft stool that passes promptly and easily through your digestive tract.

Besides being an element in wheat and other whole grains, insoluble fiber is found in fruits and vegetables, usually in the outer layers, such as the skins of apples and peaches and the protective coatings of seeds and legumes. Wheat bran, which is the outer layer of each grain, is almost entirely insoluble fiber.

By creating bulk in your intestines and speeding up the passage of food, insoluble fiber provides several important health benefits. It helps reduce constipation and hemorrhoids, and it appears to help prevent diverticulosis, a condition in which your intestinal wall weakens, creating tiny pockets that can trap food and become painfully inflamed. Insoluble fiber is also associated with a reduced incidence of colon cancer, possibly because it increases the excretion of bile acids. Consuming foods rich in insoluble fiber also helps keep your weight down. Not only does fiber fill you up without adding calories, but "chewy," fibrous foods tend to take longer to consume than sweet or fatty foods.

Soluble fiber consists of pectins and gums found in the inside sections of legumes, nuts, fruits and vegetables, as well as in the brans and kernels of oats, barley, rice and rye. This type of fiber does not appear to speed your digestion of food; rather, it works chemically to affect certain metabolic processes. For example, soluble fiber binds fatty compounds and transports them out of your body to lower overall cholesterol levels. As it breaks down, the fiber produces substances that also inhibit your production of cholesterol. Eating foods that are high in soluble fiber — oat bran, carrots, citrus fruits, apples, okra, dried beans, peas and lentils

Increasing Your Fiber Intake

It is recommended that adults consume 25 to 35 grams of dietary fiber daily, yet most Americans eat only five to 10 grams each day. To include more of this vital element in your diet, it helps to be aware of the amounts of fiber in various foods. Food companies are beginning to advertise the fiber content of their products and are also adding it to some varieties. In addition, you can increase your fiber intake by adopting the following eating habits:

◆ Eat a variety of foods. Many people think that they are getting enough fiber by simply eating some bran. However, if you use bran alone to create a high-fiber diet, you will be not get the range of benefits that different forms of fiber provide. You should have a diet that includes plenty of whole grains, fruits, vegetables and legumes. (Some of the best high-fiber foods are listed on the opposite page.)

◆ Eat fruits and vegetables raw whenever possible. Boiling, peeling or processing foods such as apples, carrots and broccoli tends to reduce their fiber content. And when you have potatoes, eat the skins, which are quite high in fiber.

◆ Do not consume all of your fiber in one meal. It may be tempting to eat a great deal of fiber at breakfast, since many cereals and whole-grain breads are excellent sources. If you eat too much fiber at one sitting, you increase the chance of having unpleasant side effects such as abdominal gas and diarrhea. Excess fiber can also limit the absorption of iron and other trace minerals.

◆ Drink plenty of fluids. Some people think that too much water with high-fiber foods can cause bloating, but this is not true. In fact, if there is not enough fluid for the fiber to absorb, it can slow or even block digestion. Water also helps you feel full without adding calories.

and barley — has been shown to reduce blood cholesterol by 6 to as much as 19 percent.

Some forms of soluble fiber also appear to affect blood sugar levels, most dramatically in diabetics. In studies of people with type-II (adult-onset) diabetes, those subjects who consumed high-fiber diets showed improved glucose tolerance and therefore were able to reduce their insulin requirements.

If you want to obtain specific benefits from fiber, you do not have to keep close track of which type of fiber you eat: Most plant foods contain both types in varying proportions. Moreover, a healthy diet should emphasize a variety of foods, not only to ensure that you get the benefits of various forms of fiber, but that your intake of other necessary nutrients is adequate.

The least effective way of adding fiber to your diet is with supplements. Not only do they tend to provide only one type of fiber, they do not provide the same benefits as the fiber that you consume in whole foods. You also lose the vitamins, minerals and energy nutrients that are part of most high-fiber foods. Finally, taking supplements can lead you to consume too much fiber too quickly. One consequence of this can be intestinal gas due to fermentation, which can result in painful stomach cramps. Because fiber absorbs water, eating excessive amounts can also cause dehydration. And fiber binds with iron and other trace minerals, so that too much fiber can limit the absorption of these nutrients. The recommendations in the box *(above)* should help ensure that you eat the correct amount of fiber.

Fitness

No matter what shape you want to be in, physical fitness requires a progressive, continuous effort to improve your endurance, strength and flexibility. Physiologists say that the health benefits of fitness do not come from the state of being fit, but from the effort to achieve it, meaning exercise.

A regular program of exercise appears to be increasingly important to combat the process of aging. Many of the problems commonly associated with aging — increased body fat, decreased muscle strength and flexibility, loss of bone mass and lower metabolism — are more accurately described as symptoms of inactivity that can be minimized or prevented with exercise. Indeed, many healthy people over 50 who exercise regularly are more fit, according to standard measures, than sedentary young people. Regular exercise can measurably improve four basic elements of physical fitness: Cardiovascular endurance, muscle strength, endurance and flexibility.

Cardiovascular endurance is usually defined as your ability to perform a vigorous activity such as running, brisk walking, cycling or swimming for an extended period of time. Indeed, it is the most vital element of fitness. To build cardiovascular endurance, you must enhance the ability of your heart and blood vessels to deliver oxygen to your muscles and improve their capacity to use the oxygen and eliminate waste products. Although your muscles can draw on quick sources of energy for short-term exertion, such as lifting a heavy weight, when the exercise lasts longer than a minute or two, they get energy from a process that requires oxygen from the blood. Such activi-

ty is called "aerobic," meaning "life with air."

With regular aerobic exercise, your heart can pump more blood, and thus deliver more oxygen with greater efficiency, and then recover more quickly after exertion. See pages 20-21 for the three-minute step test, which measures your heart's ability to recover from a period of vigorous exercise.

Regular aerobic exercise helps keep your blood pressure within normal levels, reduces the risk of heart disease and aids in weight control. There is also evidence that it can raise your "good" HDL cholesterol level. Aerobic exercise may help reduce the risk of osteoporosis and is important in the management of diabetes.

Some research has also shown that an aerobic exercise program can have a wide range of psychological benefits that includes improved self-esteem, lessened anxiety and relief from depression. In addition, exercisers often report that they are able to cope with stress better than sedentary people.

Muscular strength is the force that a muscle produces in one all-out effort. Muscle endurance refers to the ability to perform repeated muscular contractions in quick succession: for example, doing 20 push-ups in a minute. Although muscle endurance does require strength, it is not a single all-out effort. The key to increasing endurance is building up your exercise repetition, working at a moderate level of exertion.

Everyone should have both muscle strength and endurance. Well-toned muscles are attractive, help you maintain good posture and prevent injuries. You can build

Getting Started

The American College of Sports Medicine (ACSM) suggests that an aerobic exercise program consists of 15- to 60-minute sessions of continuous, vigorous exercise three to five days a week. Any activity is acceptable as long as it can be maintained continually and utilizes your leg muscles. Examples include running, brisk walking, swimming, cycling, rowing, cross-country skiing, and rope jumping. The exercise must be intense enough to raise your heart rate to its training zone, which can be computed as 65 to 85 percent of your age-predicted maximum (220 minus your age). Stop-and-go sports such as tennis or baseball will not keep your heart rate high enough to qualify as aerobic activities.

◆ If you are over 45 and have not exercised regularly in a year or more, or if you are any age and have any coronary artery disease risk factors (high blood pressure or heart disease in your family, for instance), you should consult with your physician before engaging in strenuous exercise.

◆ As part of a beginning program, aim for three 30-minute workouts a week, each with a five-minute warm-up, a 20-minute training session and a five-minute cool-down. Give yourself at least 24 hours of recovery between each exercise day.

◆ Gradually work up to an optimal level for aerobic training, which consists of four weekly workouts of 40 or more minutes each, including five minutes of warm-ups and five minutes of cool-downs. Experiment by cutting back on your exercise times but working out an extra day, for instance. Or do "hard-easy" workouts: Shorten the duration but increase the intensity of your routine on one day while cutting back on the intensity and lengthening the duration the next.

◆ Although occasional minor aches and pains are inevitable results of any exercise program, never "run through" the pain of an injury. Most injuries can be averted by wearing appropriate shoes (see page 91 for tips on choosing the right shoe) and avoiding training errors such as trying to do too much too soon. Always start gradually and increase the duration or intensity of your workouts only by about 10 percent a week. For more information on injury prevention and treatment, see pages 120-121.

strength and endurance through progressive-resistance training, which requires applying resistance to various body movements. The weights are heavy enough to make you contract your muscles at tensions close to maximum, and are progressively increased to stimulate them to develop. In a typical progressive-resistance weight-training program, you lift weights that are 75 to 85 percent of your maximum ability for three sets of 10 to 15 repetitions. This is done for each muscle group. To allow your muscles to recover properly, you should lift weights no more than every other day. If you train more than that, your muscles will not have time to recuperate.

Flexibility is the ability of your joints to move through their full range of motion. Since short, tight muscles are more likely to be pulled, good flexibility and regular stretching protect your muscles against injury. Athletes often stretch after intense bouts of exercise to relieve muscle soreness. Also, stretching pelvic muscles has been shown to alleviate menstrual cramps.

To improve your flexibility, carefully warm up by jogging in place or cycling on an exercise bike. Then perform slow, static stretches until you feel a mildly uncomfortable pulling sensation—but not pain—in the center of your muscle. Hold the stretch for 10 to 30 seconds, relax and then repeat it. Be sure not to bounce your limbs in exaggerated movements or force your stretches in any way, which could cause an injury.

Food Additives

Food additives have existed for thousands of years, at least since the discovery that salt preserved meat and fish. And they are not likely to disappear, since Americans now depend on an ever-increasing variety of convenience foods that require additives.

Although some of these substances offer indisputable health benefits, such as protection from deadly botulin poisoning, most additives are used solely to make foods more attractive and palatable. Surveys reveal that consumers are highly concerned about chemical additives. Yet, in spite of this concern, the average American eats between five and 10 pounds of chemical additives in foods annually, and the figure continues to increase.

Despite the public's heightened awareness in recent years about the artificial sweetener cyclamate, a plant-growth regulator called Alar and other approved substances that were shown to cause cancer in animals, the food supply in the United States is more closely scrutinized and additives more strictly regulated than ever before. Food additives are extensively studied and regulated, primarily by the federal Food and Drug Administration (FDA).

Since 1958, manufacturers of foods have had to prove the safety of any new additive; before that, the burden was on the government to prove the health hazards of a substance. However, about 700 additives have been exempted from testing because of their long history of use without any harmful effects. These additives are referred to as "generally recognized as safe" (GRAS). Unfortunately, many of the most widely used and controversial additives are on the GRAS list, which authorizes their use.

The FDA has been re-evaluating all GRAS substances and has banned or restricted the use of some of them. Meanwhile, there is still controversy surrounding certain artificial colors and preservatives on the GRAS list.

The most restrictive legislation states that substances shown to cause cancer in animals or humans may not be added to foods in any amount. Food producers argue against this rule on the grounds that, in some cases, the cancer risk is minuscule, or that any risk is outweighed by the benefits provided by the additive. The small risk of cancer from ingesting a certain preservative, for instance, may be offset by eliminating a greater risk of contracting botulism. Nitrites — weak carcinogens that are still on the market — are in this category.

Most of the estimated 3,000 compounds deliberately added to foods fall into one of the categories shown in the additives chart at right. However, there may be as many as 10,000 "indirect" additives, which are detectable substances that are found or added to foods during packaging, storing or processing.

The best way to reduce your consumption of additives is to restrict your intake of refined or convenience foods, including junk foods. Instead, eat fresh or minimally processed foods. Read food labels carefully (but keep in mind that additives are not always listed), and limit your intake of foods that have artificial colors. (See pages 88-89 for information about food labels.) It is also important to eat a variety of foods, since this limits your exposure to any one potentially harmful additive.

Guide to Food Additives

TYPE	FUNCTION	USE	COMMENTS
Preservatives: *Nitrates, nitrites, BHA, BHT, sulfites, benzoic acid, ascorbic acid, calcium propionate*	Retard spoilage from bacteria, fungi, molds; keep fats and oils from turning rancid; delay discoloration, as in cut fruit	Most processed or prepared foods	Sulfites can cause allergic reactions, especially in asthmatics. Nitrates and nitrites have induced cancer in animals; limit intake of cured meats. BHT and BHA are under review.
Nutrients: *Vitamins, minerals*	Replace nutrients lost in processing, improve nutritive value of foods	Processed cereals, flour, rice, milk, margarine, salt	Most vitamins are artificially synthesized but are chemically identical to natural substances.

TO INCREASE APPEAL

TYPE	FUNCTION	USE	COMMENTS
Colors: *Annatto, carotene, caramel, fruit juice, chlorophyll, saffron, synthetic colors*	Improve appearance by giving food an appetizing, characteristic color	Used in all kinds of processed foods	Can conceal omission of an ingredient or mask poor quality. Synthetic dyes are widely used; their safety is under review. Yellow no. 5 (tartrazine) must be listed on labels because of allergic reactions.
Flavors: *Vanilla, spices, seasonings, artificial flavors*	Improve taste; restore flavor lost in processing	Baked goods, soft drinks and many other products	Largest category of additives. Can be listed on labels in general terms such as natural or artificial flavors or spices.
Flavor enhancers: *MSG, hydrolyzed vegetable protein, maltol*	Modify taste or aroma of food	Oriental foods, soup mixes, canned vegetables, gravies	MSG causes allergic reactions in some people. Hydrolyzed vegetable protein can produce MSG when heated and combined with salt.
Sweeteners: *Natural sugars (fructose, corn syrup), artificial sweeteners (saccharin, aspartame)*	Provide sweetness; sugar is also a common preservative.	Baked goods, candy, soft drinks, jams and many processed foods	Many consumers are concerned about artificial sweeteners because of the controversy surrounding saccharin and the banning of cyclamates in 1970. Aspartame's safety is under review.

TO AID IN PROCESSING

TYPE	FUNCTION	USE	COMMENTS
Emulsifiers (mixers): *Lecithin, mono/diglycerides, polysorbates*	Keep liquid particles evenly mixed and homogenous	Ice cream, baked goods, margarine, dressings, gelatin	Help disperse oils and flavors, as in mayonnaise and peanut butter. Many come from natural sources.
Stabilizers, thickeners, texturizers: *Gums, modified starch, pectin, cellulose, carrageenan*	Improve consistency and provide texture	Most prepared desserts, sauces, jams and jellies, baked goods, soups	Many are natural carbohydrates that absorb water in foods. They affect "mouth feel" of foods, for instance, by preventing ice crystals from forming in ice cream.
pH control agents: *Citric acid, acetic acid, alkalis, buffers*	Control acidity or alkalinity, affecting texture and taste	Soft drinks, dairy products, canned vegetables, fruit products, baked goods	Also used to prevent botulism in low-acid canned goods such as beets. Some acids help dough rise.

Food Labels

With a growing concern about the potential dangers of food additives and the trend toward low-fat, low-salt diets, more people are carefully scrutinizing food labels. However, food labels do not always tell the whole truth; they frequently obscure as much as they reveal.

While many labels display no nutritional or ingredient information, others provide misleading indications. For instance, a food labeled "sugar-free" or "light" can be laden with calories; one with "no salt added" can be packed with sodium; and a "natural" food can contain a vast array of artificial ingredients.

There are presently about 300 foods — from ice cream to mayonnaise — that are not required to list ingredients or nutrients because they are made according to legally standardized recipes. All other foods must have a list of ingredients on their labels, but the lists can be misleading. Most food colors, flavors and spices do not have to be listed by name. Instead, general terms such as "artificial and natural flavors" can

Commonly Misunderstood Terms

DIET, DIETETIC

Means that a product is either a reduced-calorie or a low-calorie food (see below). These terms can also appear on the labels of products that are used for special dietary purposes.

HEALTH FOOD

This term does not have a legal definition. It is frequently used in a misleading way, claiming that a certain food can promote health.

LEAN

Indicates that a product is no more than 10 percent fat by weight. An exception to this definition is "lean" ground beef, which may contain as much as 30 percent fat by weight in most states. "Extra lean" must be no more than 5 percent fat. If "lean" is used as part of a brand name to indicate that a product may be helpful in reducing weight, the product is required to display a nutrition label.

LIGHT, LITE

These words are virtually meaningless. If "light" refers to reduced calories, full nutrition information must be provided. But "light" can also refer to pale color, low sodium or fat, taste, fluffy texture or reduced alcohol content, as in "light" beer. When applied to processed meats, "light" means that products have at least 25 percent less fat than usual.

LOW CALORIE

A "low-calorie" food must have 40 calories or less per serving and less than .4 calories per gram. A salad dressing with 35 calories per tablespoon may appear to be low calorie because of its small serving size, but it would not qualify since it contains more than .4 calories per gram. This term cannot be used on the label of a food that is naturally low in calories, such as mushrooms.

LOW SALT

Refers to products made with less salt than the usual variety of the same product. However, people limiting their sodium intake should read labels carefully because a food low in salt is not necessarily low in sodium. Salt contains sodium, but many other ingredients contain sodium as well.

LOW SODIUM

Means a product contains 140 milligrams or less of sodium per serving, equivalent to approximately a 1/14 teaspoon of salt.

NATURAL

When applied to meat or poultry, "natural" means the food is minimally processed and free of artificial colors, flavors, preservatives and synthetic ingredients. For other foods, "natural" has no legal meaning. Many "natural" foods are highly processed, packed with fat and sugar and loaded with preservatives. Carbonated soft drinks, beer and potato chips are among the many products that are "natural."

be listed on the label. If you are allergic to certain food colors, flavors or spices and wish to avoid them, you must write to the food manufacturers to find out which ones are used in a particular product.

Food labels also tell little about fat and cholesterol content. A nutritional label must list how many grams of fat are in a serving, but a breakdown of the fats into unsaturated and saturated fatty acids is optional. A label indicating the cholesterol content of a food is also optional, unless a specific claim is made about it.

Fortunately, many important label regulations exist in the United States. If a product regulated by the FDA makes nutritional claims (such as "high in iron"), contains added nutrients or is intended for special dietary uses, it must display complete nutritional information on its label to substantiate the claims. Ingredients must be listed in descending order according to weight, although this does not reveal how much of any ingredient is actually used. To help you with some of the terms on food labels, see the glossary *(below)*.

NATURALLY FLAVORED

A "natural flavor" must come from a juice, oil, leaf, herb, root, spice or other natural source. However, a product containing "all natural flavor" may still contain artificial colors and preservatives.

NO CHOLESTEROL

Although a food may not contain cholesterol, which occurs only in animal products, it may still contain saturated fat, which raises the level of blood cholesterol even more than dietary cholesterol. Coconut oil and palm oil, for example, are highly saturated, but do not contain cholesterol.

ORGANIC

Manufacturers may put this term on labels without any guidelines since it has not been legally defined. However, the U.S. Department of Agriculture does not permit "organic" to appear on poultry or meat products. "Organic" is popularly defined as a food or nutrient produced without pesticides, additives or chemical fertilizers. "Organic" products are frequently more expensive than the regular variety of the same product, and are, in some cases, unsafe to use.

REDUCED CALORIES

Foods with this label must have at least one-third fewer calories than the regular version. The calorie content per serving of both the "reduced-calorie" food and the food with which it is being compared must be shown on the label.

SODIUM-FREE

This term means that a product must contain fewer than 5 milligrams of sodium per serving.

SUGAR-FREE, SUGARLESS

These products contain no sucrose (table sugar) but they may have other types of sweeteners, such as fructose, honey, corn syrup, or sorbitol, all of which may contain as many calories as sucrose. Thus, "sugar-free" and "sugarless" foods may still be high in calories.

Foot Care

Each foot is an interlocking network of 20 muscles, 28 bones and 112 ligaments structurally similar to your hand. All together, your hands and feet contain half the bones in your body. Although related in many respects, your hands and feet, of course, perform vastly different tasks: Your hands are designed for manipulation, while your feet are engineered for support of your body.

Healthy feet are indispensable for an active life. Structured like arched bridges to efficiently support great weight and stress, your feet can absorb the repeated shock of your locomotion. They alternately absorb impact as you walk and run, and then, like springs, they return the energy for propulsion.

For all their importance, however, your feet are neglected too often, or even abused until there is a problem that may cause discomfort or disfigurement. Four out of five adults have painful feet, a condition that too many people merely accept as a fact of life.

Some conditions, such as obesity, poor circulation, arthritis, and diabetes, can cause or exacerbate foot problems. But much everyday foot discomfort stems from ill-fitting shoes, socks and stockings, or from foot gear that is not appropriate for an activity. Most common types of foot pain, in fact, are preventable or can be treated effectively without professional help. If a medical problem is the cause of your foot pain, you should consult either an orthopedist, a physician certified in the care of bone and joint disorders, or a podiatrist, a foot specialist who can perform minor surgery and prescribe medication if necessary.

Shoes

Your shoes can either be your best protection against foot pain or the direct cause of your discomfort. When buying shoes, remember that your foot size can change as you age, gain or lose weight, alter your lifestyle — such as an increase in your exercise habits — and even change with the time of day.

Always have your foot measured, and try on more than one size on each foot for comparison. Buy shoes at midday or later, when your feet have widened slightly with activity. Make sure that the area at the widest part of your foot has adequate room in the shoe, and allow at least a half inch of space in front of the tip of your big toe. Never buy shoes that have to be broken in; they should be comfortable immediately. See the box (opposite) for tips when choosing athletic shoes.

Because stylish shoes for women often have high heels and pointed toes, and are too narrow and unstable, they have far more foot and ankle problems than men. If you have high heels, wear them for special occasions. Wear comfortable walking shoes whenever you can. Remember to replace worn heels and discard worn-out shoes. Uneven heels can decrease foot stability and place undue stress on your muscles and joints.

Athlete's Foot

Cracking, blistering and peeling skin, and intense itching between your toes, are frequent symptoms of athlete's foot. Almost one-third of Americans suffer this malady, making it the nation's number-one skin prob-lem. Athlete's foot is really a collection of diseases, ranging from a fungus infection to allergic reactions to perspiration, dyes or drugs. Obesity, diabetes and arthritis can contribute to athlete's foot. A doctor may prescribe antifungal medications. For the best prevention, wash your feet daily, wear clean, dry socks and open, ventilated shoes as much as possible, and avoid rubber- or plastic-soled shoes, which increase foot perspiration. Expose your feet to the air and sunlight whenever possible.

Blisters, Corns and Calluses

Friction or pressure from ill-fitting shoes, socks or stockings — or not wearing socks at all — causes blisters. They are also the most common athletic injuries, usually caused by friction between ill-fitting socks and your feet. To a avoid them, wear clean, seamless socks and apply petroleum jelly to portions of your feet that may be susceptible to friction.

To treat a blister that is a half-inch in diameter or smaller, make sure the area is clean. Cover it with a thin foam pad with a hole in the center, or with a patch of adhesive tape. Avoid breaking the blister. You can also leave the area uncovered and go barefoot indoors. For larger blisters, or for those that break, wash the area and cover it with a light bandage. You should see a physician if the blister becomes infected.

Corns and calluses result from pressure and chafing, often from tight shoes. Corns are thickened skin, usually on your toes. Hard corns can appear on your little toe, while soft corns will appear on the webs

Choosing the Right Shoe

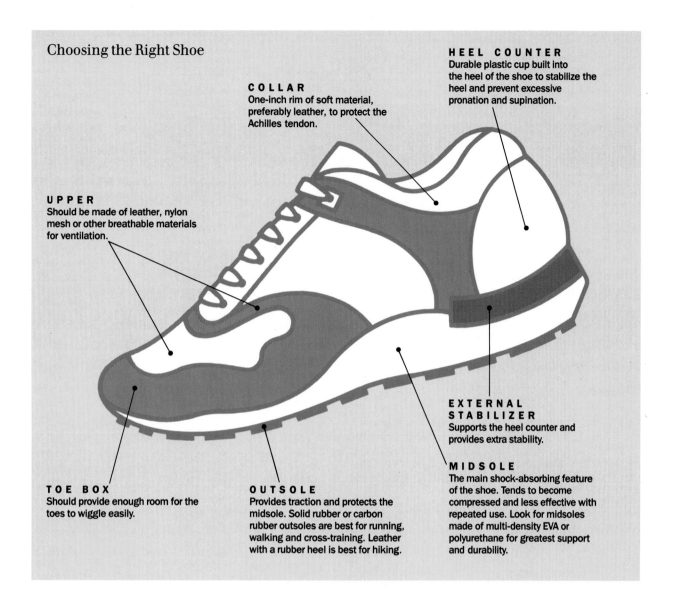

HEEL COUNTER
Durable plastic cup built into the heel of the shoe to stabilize the heel and prevent excessive pronation and supination.

COLLAR
One-inch rim of soft material, preferably leather, to protect the Achilles tendon.

UPPER
Should be made of leather, nylon mesh or other breathable materials for ventilation.

TOE BOX
Should provide enough room for the toes to wiggle easily.

OUTSOLE
Provides traction and protects the midsole. Solid rubber or carbon rubber outsoles are best for running, walking and cross-training. Leather with a rubber heel is best for hiking.

EXTERNAL STABILIZER
Supports the heel counter and provides extra stability.

MIDSOLE
The main shock-absorbing feature of the shoe. Tends to become compressed and less effective with repeated use. Look for midsoles made of multi-density EVA or polyurethane for greatest support and durability.

between your toes. Calluses often form on or around your heel or on the ball of your foot. Most calluses are natural barriers that prevent injuries to underlying soft tissues. When they are no longer needed, they usually soften and peel off. Some calluses, however, turn hard and dry and the area surrounding them becomes red and inflamed.

The best way to treat troublesome hard corns and calluses is to soak your foot in warm water until your skin softens, then gently rub it with a pumice stone. While it may take several treatments to remove a corn or callus, do not rub it raw. If self-treatment does not work, consult a doctor. After removing the corn or callus, cover the area with a light pad or bandage. Avoid treatments with salicylic acid, because it can burn your skin and cause infection.

Your feet were made for walking, and walking regularly will help keep them in good condition. It will improve the circulation to your legs and feet and reduce your risk of arthritis and obesity, two major contributors to foot problems.

For many sports and activities, well-fitting shoes are crucial to help prevent injuries. The right shoes provide you with proper support and shock absorption and prevent excessive pronation or supination — inward or outward rolling of your feet. Although exercise shoes come in a wide array of options and styles, the illustration above features most of the elements you should look for when purchasing many types of athletic shoes.

Headaches

Almost everyone gets an occasional headache. Usually, headaches are annoyances triggered by colds, stress, fatigue or simply being in a smoky room, and they are easily relieved by a simple pain reliever. But for some 12 to 20 million Americans, headaches are severe, chronic problems that require careful medical evaluation and treatment supervision.

While there are numerous types of headaches, they can all be divided into three main categories: muscle-contraction, or tension, headaches; vascular types associated with abnormal dilation or constriction of blood vessels in your brain; and organic headaches that are symptoms of other health problems. The chart at right will help you to distinguish among the three most common types of nonorganic headaches.

Until recently, 80 to 90 percent of all headaches were blamed on muscle contractions, which result from tension that causes your head and neck muscles to tighten, putting pressure on nerves and blood vessels. However, researchers have discovered that many people who presumably had muscular-contraction headaches actually did not exhibit any abnormal muscle tension. These findings led specialists to believe that vascular headaches account for a greater percentage of headaches than they had thought previously.

Vascular headaches produce severe and throbbing pain, possibly because of blood pulsing through your enlarged cerebral blood vessels. The most severe vascular headaches are migraines and clusters, although some other types, such as headaches accompanying hangovers or following physical exertion, are also vascular in origin. Although migraines and clusters are believed to be the result of similar abnormal blood flow, their symptoms and patterns of occurrence vary considerably.

Migraines have genetic components: If someone in your family suffers from migraines, your chances of experiencing them increase; and 70 percent of victims are women. Female migraine sufferers often have more frequent and severe attacks around menstruation time, but incidences decrease during pregnancy and after menopause. Also, oral contraceptives may increase the onset of migraines. Such patterns as these have led scientists to examine a possible connection between hormones and migraines.

Research has also found a possible biochemical factor in migraines: Sufferers often have abnormally high levels of certain brain chemicals that may affect the dilation and contraction of blood vessels. Perhaps because of damage to the optic nerves that results from reduced blood flow, one recent study showed that 35 percent of migraine sufferers experience peripheral-vision impairment.

In contrast to migraines, which occur sporadically, cluster headaches strike in a series: The victim has several severe headaches a day, possibly for weeks at a time. However, in most cases, there are periods of remission between clusters. And they are vastly more common among men than women.

Organic headaches are frequently symptoms of underlying disorders. By far the most common disease associated with headaches is high blood pressure; indeed, headaches are often the only symptoms. If you suffer from frequent headaches,

---

Strenuous exertion sometimes triggers exercise-induced headaches. If you suffer occasional headaches during or immediately after exercise, you can often prevent them by warming up for 25 minutes prior to exercise. You can also take ibuprofen and cut back on your training, then slowly build back up again. Of course, if you suffer chronic or severe headaches, whether or not they are associated with exercise, consult your doctor.

What Kind of Headache Is It?

	TENSION	MIGRAINE	CLUSTER
Who gets them	Anyone	Tendency to run in families; seven times as many women afflicted as men; onset usually in adolescence or early adulthood	85 percent of victims are men, usually between the ages of 20 and 60; average age of onset is 40
Symptoms	Frontal, bandlike or generalized pain aggravated by head movement; may be accompanied by muscle spasms in neck and upper back	Severe, throbbing pain that commonly begins in the eyes and spreads to either one or both sides of the head; nausea and vomiting often occur; pain is aggravated by light and sound; may be preceded by a visual aura, such as flashing lights or jagged lines, language disturbances or motor weakness	Abrupt onset of severe, steady, one-sided pain usually localized around an eye; significant flushing and nasal congestion on affected side
Frequency	Variable	Can occur weekly or only once or twice yearly	Several times daily for a period of weeks or months
Duration	Usually several hours	Usually several hours to one day	Less than three hours
Triggers	Anxiety, noise, fatigue, depression or environmental irritants	Caused by abnormal dilation and constriction of blood vessels in the brain, migraines can be triggered by foods containing MSG, nitrites or tyramine, a chemical found in foods such as red wine and ripe cheese; certain odors, oral contraceptives, alcohol, menstruation, hunger, fatigue, hypertension, stress or anxiety	Like migraines, cluster headaches are due to dilation and constriction of blood vessels in the brain; alcohol and/or smoking frequently precipitate an attack

have your blood pressure checked, especially if you are over 40.

A more rare cause of headaches is a brain tumor. In fact, headaches associated with brain tumors are found in less than half of one percent of all those who seek treatment for headaches. However, the sudden onset of a severe headache if you rarely had them previously might signify a serious disorder, such as a cerebral aneurysm, and should prompt a visit to your doctor.

Headaches that occur after a mild blow to the head, which may result during a game of football or other contact sport, are fairly common. People who experience recurrent headaches or other symptoms such as dizziness should be examined by a doctor.

Treatments for headaches largely depend on which types you suffer from and their frequency. In some cases, you must consult your physician. There are two basic categories of medicines: The first is abortive drugs — analgesics like aspirin, acetaminophen and ibuprofen; as well as narcotics like codeine and Demerol — which relieve pain and other symptoms after an attack. The second category consists of prophylactic drugs — preventive daily medication that blocks the causes of vascular headaches and eliminates the onset of frequent attacks.

Nondrug treatments are often effective for many people, since side effects are avoided. Hot or cold pads placed around your neck or head, or hot baths may relieve some muscle-contraction headaches. Massaging your forehead, temples, neck and shoulders is another treatment. Running cold water over your head to constrict swollen blood vessels may alleviate a vascular headache; you can also put your hands in hot water, which draws blood to them, possibly relieving pressure in your head. Finally, relaxation techniques such as exercise, meditation, Yoga and biofeedback have all provided some relief to headache sufferers.

Heat and Cold

Most active people go outdoors in all sorts of weather. They hike in the heat of summer, run in the rain or cross-country ski on winter nights. While exercising in different weather conditions can be exhilarating, it is important to be aware of the dangers of heat and cold. Many problems can be avoided easily by taking a few simple precautions. The first step in both hot and cold weather is to make sure that you are properly conditioned to perform an activity. While certain people are at high risk of being affected by extreme weather conditions — children, older people and those who are ill or out of shape — even highly trained athletes are susceptible to the elements.

Hyperthermia

No other mammal is as uniquely suited to physical exertion on hot days as humans. While many other mammals must pant to stay cool, humans depend on sweat evaporation to reduce body temperature. Indeed, humans can sweat as much as four quarts an hour. But overconfidence in your body's ability to cool itself rapidly can lead to trouble.

Heat production in exercising muscles can be 15 to 20 times that of muscles at rest. In hot weather, that excess heat must be dissipated by sweat to prevent a dangerous rise in body temperature called hyperthermia. However, when the relative humidity increases, the air becomes more saturated with water vapor, reducing the effectiveness of sweat evaporation to cool you down. When the humidity rises over 75 percent, sweat production begins to lose its

effectiveness; when it reaches 100 percent, evaporation stops completely. The accumulation of sweat on your skin may also close your sweat ducts, thus allowing your skin to become hot and dry. Without sweat evaporation, your body temperature can increase to cause heatstroke, permanent injury or even death.

Hyperthermia is also possible in arid climates, where sweat can evaporate so rapidly that you may lose a tremendous amount of fluid before you realize it. Dehydration can occur in a short time or develop over several days. If you exercise under these conditions and do not drink fluids, your body will not be able to produce enough sweat to cool itself. If you are not accustomed to a hot climate, monitor your weight regularly, since rapid losses indicate dehydration.

The best way to avoid hyperthermia is to drink plenty of fluids, dress properly and avoid exercising when it is hot and humid. On sunny summer days, avoid strenuous exercise between the hours of 10 a.m. and 2 p.m., when the sun is strongest.

Hypothermia

Hypothermia — a severe drop in body temperature — can occur if you are exposed to extremely cold temperatures or if your skin becomes wet, causing you to lose body heat very rapidly.

While exercise increases your metabolism and reduces your risk of hypothermia, frostbite or other cold-weather injuries, it is important to guard against the dangers of hypothermia by dressing properly and staying dry. Drink fluids even in cold weather, since dehydration can also

exacerbate hypothermia. When exposed to wind and extreme cold, cover your ears and nose. Wear mittens instead of gloves to protect your fingers, and wear wool socks in your boots to wick away sweat. Also, make sure that your shoes and socks are not so tight that they constrict the flow of blood to your toes; wiggle them frequently, and periodically take your feet out of your shoes or boots for a few moments to increase blood circulation.

One mistake that many people make when exercising in the cold is to overdress, which can cause your clothes to become damp with sweat, and result in a risk of hypothermia once you stop. While cross-country skiing, for example, you need one-sixth the thermal protection you need when you stop to rest. To avoid overheating and then becoming cold when you stop or slow down, layer your clothing so that you can easily remove articles when you are active and creating a significant amount of body heat, and then bundle yourself up again when you stop to rest.

People are in particular danger of hypothermia after sustaining an injury, if they are unconscious, in shock, or not able to produce body heat. In such cases, hypothermia will increase the risk of frostbite. For immediate care, take a person suffering from hypothermia to a warm room and, if he is conscious, give him warm liquids to drink and cover him with blankets. If you are in the woods, put the victim in a sleeping bag and transport him to safety as soon as possible. Get medical attention immediately. The charts (opposite) give the warning signs and some tips to avoid both heat- and cold-related injuries.

HYPOTHERMIA

You are at risk if you are:

- *Under 15 or over 40*
- *Thin*
- *Sick or injured*
- *Wet*
- *Under the influence of alcohol or drugs*
- *A smoker*

Warning signs:

- *Muscle weakness*
- *Drowsiness*
- *Confusion*
- *Clumsiness*
- *Depressed heart rate and breathing*
- *Pale, numb patches of skin indicating frostbite*

Prevention tips:

- *Wear layers of clothing*
- *Wear gloves or mittens*
- *Wear a hat*
- *Stay dry*
- *Avoid exhaustion*
- *Do not risk getting lost*

HYPERTHERMIA

You are at risk if you are:

- *Under 15 or over 40*
- *Obese*
- *Sick*
- *Dehydrated*
- *Unaccustomed to heat*
- *In poor physical condition*

Warning signs:

- *Headache*
- *Excessive sweating*
- *Inability to sweat*
- *Muscle cramps*
- *Dizziness*
- *Confusion*
- *Chills*
- *Nausea*

Prevention tips:

- *Drink plenty of water*
- *Avoid heavy exercise in hot and humid weather*

Home Environment

Traditionally, your home is considered a haven that protects you from the dangers of the outside world. However, environmental toxins are being found in many households. Studies have shown that the public health risk of cancer from exposure to chemicals in household materials like solvents and paint strippers is greater than that from toxic waste dumps.

Basically, household contaminants are of two categories: those that are used in construction, such as asbestos for fireproofing and formaldehyde for insulation, and those that are brought in or find their way into your home, such as radon, combustion gases and contaminated water. According to estimates by the Environmental Protection Agency (EPA), about 10 percent of all homes have potentially life-threatening levels of radon gas, which is responsible for 20,000 cancer deaths each year.

Since many toxins cannot be smelled, seen or tasted, detecting and removing them often require the services of a specialist. Before hiring any detection or removal company, carefully evaluate its reputation and check references. Some companies, such as those engaged in asbestos detection and removal, are certified by the EPA; others, such as testers for radon, are state-certified.

You can also cut down on pollutants by trying not to bring them into your home. Make sure that you purchase formaldehyde-free building products, for example. If you are buying a new home, have a professional evaluate the building site for radon levels and the building materials that are used.

Household Pollutants

	DESCRIPTION
Asbestos	Fibrous mineral formerly used in insulation, fire- and soundproofing, as well as in paint and joint compounds
Combustion gases	Gaseous by-products of fuel-burning appliances, such as carbon monoxide or dioxide or hydrogen cyanide
Formaldehyde	Common gas present in resins of most particleboard, plywood and wood paneling; insulation; adhesives of carpeting and wallpaper; permanent-press clothing; toothpaste
Radon	Radioactive gas produced by the decay of uranium in soil and rocks; radon passes through spots directly accessible to soil, such as drainpipes or cracks in the foundation and basement floor. It may also be present in tap water.
Water contamination	38 million Americans drink lead-tainted water through local or household pipes. Pesticide residues, carcinogenic by-products of chlorine and other carcinogens are also present in much of the water supply. Well water may be tainted with bacteria.

RISK	POTENTIAL DANGER	ELIMINATION
Inhalation of asbestos fibers can cause asbestosis, a fatal lung disease, or cancer of the lungs, stomach and chest.	Your home may contain asbestos if it was built or remodeled between 1920-1970. Have it inspected by an EPA-certified asbestos-detection company. If it is present and flaking or crumbling, or if you renovate, it should be removed. Intact asbestos, such as pipe insulation, can be contained by wrapping the pipes with duct tape.	Removal should be done by professionals. Many states issue asbestos-removal licenses; if possible, locate a licensed company. Otherwise, check references carefully.
Buildup can cause chronic bronchitis, nausea, headaches, dizziness and fatigue.	Gas appliances, such as furnaces, wood-burning stoves and gas ranges, can discharge excessive gas if malfunctioning. Check the pilot light and burner flames on your gas range; they should be blue, not yellow. Have furnaces and appliances inspected regularly.	Clean chimneys annually. Purchase a ventilation hood for your gas range that expels gas outside; hood fans are ineffective, since they recirculate gaseous air. When buying a new range, opt for an electric or spark-ignited model. Never use a gas oven for household heating.
Can cause chronic respiratory problems, dizziness, rashes, nausea and lethargy, and asthma attacks. Has been linked to nasal cancer in animals.	Highest levels of gas are emitted when products are new, so newer homes are more likely to be contaminated. A home-test kit can determine if levels are unsafe.	Keep your home well ventilated. If tests show unsafe levels, apply epoxy sealer to particleboard, fiberboard and plywood. Also, common houseplants absorb formaldehyde. Ask for low-formaldehyde or formaldehyde-free wood and adhesives.
Inhaled radon is the second major cause of lung cancer in the U.S.; the EPA estimates that unsafe radon levels may be a factor in 9 percent of lung cancer deaths annually. The danger of radon is greatly compounded by smoking.	According to EPA estimates, 10 percent of homes in the U.S. have dangerously high levels of radon. Levels are more likely to be high if you have an unfinished basement with cracks or openings in floor and walls, an open sump pump or airtight, energy-efficient construction. Test your home with an EPA-approved alpha-tract detector. Charcoal canisters, another testing method, are less accurate; however, they can be good for preliminary screening.	If levels are unsafe, seal cracks in foundation walls and basement floors, improve ventilation with ceiling fans and keep vents open on both sides of the house. You might need to install a special ventilation system.
High consumption of lead can cause miscarriage or neurological damage in fetuses, learning disabilities in children and hypertension in adults. Other contaminants cause cancer. Bacteria can cause intestinal problems and other illnesses.	Local water suppliers can test your tap water, or can help you find a lab that will analyze it from a home-testing kit.	Running cold water from faucets for three minutes each morning will help to flush out lead. Since lead is more soluble in hot water, use cold tap water for cooking. A water purifier can eliminate much of the lead and other contaminants. Consider installing new, nonlead pipes. Have your well inspected for a cracked casing if you have harmful water bacteria.

Household Safety

Household accidents cause approximately 23,000 deaths and more than 3.5 million serious injuries annually, according to recent studies. While it may be impossible to make your household 100 percent safe, you can easily create a relatively hazard-free environment. Start by taking a room-by-room tour of your house, then implement the precautions where applicable.

Kitchens

Make sure the floor covering is made of nonslip material, such as linoleum, which provides traction, and use nonskid waxes.

To help ensure that children do not burn themselves on the stove, keep pot handles pointed toward the back of the stove, but not directly over the burners. Electric appliances should be kept away from direct heat, and when they are not in use, it is safest to keep them unplugged.

Poisonings can occur in the kitchen, especially if children have access to household cleaners. To reduce this risk, keep cleaning supplies in a safe place with childproof latches on the doors. Store cleaning fluids and any other poisonous substances in their original containers, which should be labeled clearly. (For information about how to treat a poisoned victim, see page 141.) For easy accessibility, keep a first-aid box in the kitchen. (See page 136 for tips on stocking a first-aid kit.)

Bathrooms

Electrical sockets should be insulated and plugs installed safely away from water. Most new homes have special circuit breakers in the electrical sockets near the sink. If you do not have these safety devices, inexpensive fixtures can be easily installed. To avoid slipping on wet floors, place a bath mat with a nonslip, rubberized bottom next to the tub and shower; in the tub, a rubber mat is essential to reduce the chance of falling. In 1988, more than 111,000 people reported injuries as a result of slipping in bathtubs and shower stalls. To help move in and out of the tub, securely fasten guard rails to the wall.

Never let young children bathe unattended. About 350 drownings occur every year in the bathtub. To avoid scalding, always test the water before placing a child in the tub.

Wiring

Many homes, particularly older ones, do not have enough electrical outlets. Extension cords can overload the electrical system in your home. Signs of overloaded circuits are frequently blown fuses or tripped circuit breakers, warm switches, lights that dim and television sets that flicker. If you need to use an extension cord, heavy-duty cords are the safest. However, if more outlets are necessary in a particular area of your home, consult with a licensed electrician. According to the National Board of Fire Underwriters, electrical fires often result from work done by unqualified people.

Most new homes have circuit breakers to guard against electrical overloads. When an overload occurs in a circuit breaker, a switch will automatically cut off the electricity to a certain part of your home. To restart the electricity, flick the switch back to its on position.

Older homes generally have fuse boxes. Fuses work in a similar fashion, but unlike circuit breakers they must be replaced when they blow. Be sure to replace a blown fuse only with a new one of the same capacity. To avoid electric shock, stand on a dry, nonconductive surface such as wood, using only one hand to restart the current. If the fuse blows or the circuit breaker trips repeatedly, you probably have an electrical problem such as too many appliances on a single circuit. This can lead to overheated wires in the walls and an electrical fire.

Doors and Windows

Sliding-glass doors can be dangerous if people make the mistake of walking into them. Place a decal on the glass and make sure that your door is made from tempered or laminated safety glass.

Other safety factors for homes with children are child-resistant locks and metal guards on windows. Some cities require that households with children under age 10 install window guards. If you have small children, install window guards for their protection whether they are required by law or not.

Stairs

According to the Consumer Product Safety Commission, in 1988, about 820,000 people in emergency rooms reported that their injuries were related to stairs or steps. Keep stairs

Protecting Your Home from Fires

Fire is the third-leading cause of accidental injury and death in the United States. Home fires usually begin in one of two ways: unattended cooking, resulting in stove-top or oven fires; and careless cigarette smoking, which is responsible for the most fire-related deaths in residential properties. Remember the following tips to make your home safe from fires:

◆ Install smoke detectors, and, if possible, sprinklers, in your home. Experts estimate that the proper use of smoke detectors would cut the number of fire-related deaths in half, and if detectors and sprinklers were combined, 73 percent of those who die annually in fires would be saved. Detectors should be placed near kitchens and outside bedrooms. If you or your spouse smokes, place an additional detector in your bedroom. Commercial sprinklers are particularly useful for the protection of the young, elderly and disabled who might have difficulty getting out of a fire. Alarms should be tested monthly to ensure that they are working properly.

◆ If there is no escape from the second floor, purchase or construct a fire rope or ladder; place it in an easily accessible location where it can be deployed quickly. Make sure that everyone in your home knows the most effective escape routes in the event of a fire.

◆ Have your furnace checked annually. If you smell gas from your stove or furnace, call the gas company immediately to have someone investigate a potential gas leak.

◆ Keep a fire extinguisher in a safe and convenient location in your kitchen. Salt and baking soda (but not baking powder) should also be kept handy to put out small grease fires.

◆ If you use a fireplace, keep a fire screen with fine mesh in place, have your chimney checked annually and cleaned when necessary, to guard against creosote buildup, which can lead to chimney fires.

◆ When barbecuing or building a fire in a fireplace, never pour lighter fluid or any other flammable fluid directly onto a smoldering or lit fire. For safety measures, keep a bucket of sand or a jug of water nearby.

well lit with light switches at both landings, and do not place objects on the stairs. Nonskid strips and carpeting attached to steps can be helpful in guarding against accidents. When toddlers or crawling infants are present in your home, safety gates should be in place at both the tops and bottoms of stairs.

Workshops and Garages

Keep storage areas for chemicals cool and well ventilated. Never store flammable materials indoors, and keep all flammable liquids in carefully marked, airtight cans.

Eye injuries, burns and serious wounds can occur when you use power tools. To avoid fires and power outages, always use grounded plugs and heavy-duty utility cords. Safety goggles and other appropriate protective gear are essential. Equipment should be stored where it cannot be knocked down. Keep it safely out of all children's reach.

Apart from unforeseen catastrophes, your home is generally as safe as you want it to be. Basic home precautions can protect your family, friends and neighbors as well as yourself. For information about protecting your home from the hazards of fire, see the box *(above)*.

Immunization

More than any other single medical practice, immunization has extended the life expectancy of Americans by reducing significant numbers of deaths caused by contagious illnesses. In fact, vaccination has diminished the cases of childhood diseases to less than one percent of the figure that it was just 30 years ago.

Immunization prevents diseases caused by microbes — primarily viruses — that pose serious health risks to people and do not respond to treatment effectively. It utilizes a process that occurs naturally inside your body when you contract any infectious illness, even a cold. Once you are infected by a virus, your body responds with a variety of measures, such as coughing, sneezing, developing a fever, and producing antibodies that slow down and stop the infection. Following most viral infections, your generated antibodies remain in your system to neutralize or kill the viruses should they ever appear again, without suffering through the same symptoms. In other words, you develop immunity.

Most children are infected by — and develop immunity to — about 200 common viruses, almost all of which are harmless or produce only mild and temporary illnesses. It is believed that you maintain your immunity to such viruses through persistent or recurrent benign infections. Some viruses, however, can be deadly; against these, you must be vaccinated with modified versions of the disease-causing microbes or toxins that are not strong enough to cause disease, but stimulate your system to produce antibodies. Once you are vaccinated with a particular microbe, you will be able to fend off any subsequent infection by that same virus with antibodies targeted against it. Vaccines, however, often produce only temporary immunity; after the initial vaccination, you must have booster shots or be immunized again later in life.

Through intensive vaccination programs, smallpox, which was once the most feared disease in the world, has been virtually eradicated. In the United States and other developed countries, diseases such as diphtheria, tetanus, polio and whooping cough — all of which only 50 years ago posed a major health threat, killing or crippling hundreds of thousands of children and adults — have largely been controlled.

There are potential dangers to receiving vaccinations, however. Because they introduce your body to a potential enemy, you can have unpleasant and sometimes dangerous responses. In almost all cases, the symptoms are extremely mild. For example, when a child receives the standard diphtheria, pertussis (whooping cough) and tetanus vaccine series at two months old, parents are cautioned that he or she might have a low-grade fever or be irritable for a day or two. The odds of having a more serious side effect are one in several million.

Publicity over serious adverse reactions can sometimes result in a vaccine "scare," and if immunization coverage diminishes, the disease can return in an epidemic. In response to vaccine scares, pertussis vaccinations declined in Great Britain and Japan in the late 1970s. Not surprisingly, the incidence of whooping cough claimed a tragic toll: Within two years, there were 100,000 cases and 28 deaths in Great Britain and

Should You Be Immunized?

DISEASE	PEOPLE AT RISK	VACCINE-CONFERRED IMMUNITY
Diphtheria	50 percent of adults may not be protected. Usually given in a three-dose series with tetanus in childhood; boosters are necessary every 10 years. Diphtheria is not uncommon in developing nations.	10 years
Hepatitis B	Health-care workers, homosexual males and intravenous drug users	5-10 years after three-dose series
Influenza	People over 50; diabetics; individuals with chronic illnesses of the heart, lungs or kidneys or immunosuppressant diseases such as leukemia	1 year
Measles	Anyone born after 1956 who has never been vaccinated or had the disease	Lifelong
Pneumococcal pneumonia	People over 65 or with chronic illnesses	Lifelong
Mumps	Anyone not immunized in childhood, especially adolescent and adult males, who are at higher risk for complications. Mumps is uncontrolled in many developing countries.	Lifelong
Rubella (German measles)	Unvaccinated women during childbearing years. You should not get a vaccination, however, if you are pregnant or plan to be within three months of receiving the vaccine.	Lifelong
Tetanus	Anyone not immunized in childhood or who has not received a booster in the past 10 years	10 years

13,000 cases and 41 deaths in Japan. Even in the United States, there are still between 1,500 and 2,000 cases of pertussis and four to 10 deaths from the disease each year.

Our country's wide-spread immunization policy for children — largely enforced by requiring that children be vaccinated before they enter school — successfully protects 95 percent of American children against a variety of illnesses. However, some vaccines are more important for adults than for children; without an enforced immunization policy, many adults contract unnecessary illnesses. For example, 80 percent of those at high risk for influenza do not get vaccinated annually, resulting in 10,000 deaths each year. Likewise, there are a half-million cases of pneumonia annually that could be avoided with appropriate vaccinations. Nearly half of American adults neglect to obtain their tetanus-diphtheria boosters, which are necessary every 10 years; and many of them were never immunized against measles and German measles (rubella), which can cause serious birth defects. Less than 25 percent of those at high risk for hepatitis have been immunized.

For most individuals, there is no doubt that the benefits of immunization far outweigh the risks. The chart (above) provides guidelines for which vaccinations you need. You should keep a record of all immunizations you have received from childhood on, and consult your physician about updating them if necessary. Check with your doctor if you think you are a candidate for any particular vaccine.

If you are traveling to underdeveloped countries, have the vaccinations that are recommended for those areas. You can obtain a copy of *Health Information for International Travel* from the Government Printing Office in Washington, D.C.

Medical Checkups

Getting regular checkups is an important part of preventive health care. A complete checkup, or physical, consists of a basic examination of your circulatory, digestive, respiratory, muscular and nervous systems.

A physical provides a general overview of your health, and is usually performed by your primary-care physician. This is a doctor in general or family practice or an internist who is trained to deal with most common adult health problems, and who can also refer you to an appropriate specialist if you have any serious or perplexing medical problems. Most primary-care physicians are either internists or family practitioners. (For tips on choosing a primary-care physician, see pages 70-71.)

There are four basic parts to a complete physical. On your first visit with a particular doctor, he or she will start by getting your complete medical history. The doctor will want to know about any major illnesses, accidents, hospitalizations or surgery you have had in the past, as well as any current complaints. You will probably also be asked to fill out a form that contains specific questions about your body.

Your doctor will want to obtain your social history, which includes your marital status, number of children, job, diet, exercise and health habits — all of which can have an impact on your health. He or she will inquire about any medications that you take and any allergies you might have. Finally, the doctor will ask about the health of your immediate relatives — in particular, he will want to know if there is any family history of heart disease, hypertension, cancer or diabetes.

Giving your complete medical history can make your first visit to a physician time-consuming. However, this information is one of the most valuable parts of the physical. It provides an important baseline from which your doctor can evaluate your health, determine potential problems, predict your risk factors for various conditions and suggest lifestyle improvements.

After recording the pertinent information, your doctor will conduct the actual physical examination. Like many people, you may feel uncomfortable at this point because you will need to undress, but the physician should provide you with a gown that can cover all but the area that is being examined.

Depending on your age and medical history, as well as whatever the doctor discovers during the exam, he or she may ask you to take some specific tests, such as a blood count, urinalysis or electrocardiogram.

Medical experts have established standardized schedules for particular tests and exams, as shown in the chart (opposite). Of course, your physician will recommend how frequently you should have certain exams — depending on your medical history, this might be more or less often than the established norm.

Following your exam, your physician should provide an opportunity for you to ask any questions about the checkup or your condition. He or she should also call to tell you about test results if any are pending. If you do not receive a call, it may mean that all tests were normal; however, you should feel free to call your doctor after a week to discuss anything regarding your condition that you want to inquire about specifically.

Your Examination Timetable

AGE	SEX	TEST	FREQUENCY
18-40	M/F	Complete physical	Every 4-5 years
	M/F	Blood pressure	Annually
	F	Pelvic exam, Pap smear	Annually°
	F	Breast exam	Annually
30	M/F	Exercise electrocardiogram	Every 5 years
35	M/F	Total cholesterol and high-density lipoprotein (HDL) level	Every 3 years
	M/F	Kidney function: BUN (blood, urea, nitrogen), creatinine clearance	Every 5 years
	M/F	DPT (diphtheria, pertussis, tetanus) vaccine	Every 10 years
	F	Baseline mammogram	Repeat in 5 years
40+	M/F	Complete physical	Every 3 years
	M/F	Hearing test	Every 3 years
	M/F	Visual acuity, glaucoma	Every 3 years
	M/F	Digital rectal	Annually
	F	Mammogram	Every 1-2 years
	F	Pelvic exam, Pap smear	Annually°
50	M/F	Complete physical	Every 2 years
	M/F	Baseline sigmoidoscopy (at age 40 if family history of colon-rectal disease)	Repeat in 1 year
	M/F	Stool slide test	Annually
	F	Mammogram	Annually
51	M/F	Sigmoidoscopy	Every 3 years
60	M/F	Complete physical	Annually
65	M/F	Influenza vaccine	Annually

°After a woman between the ages of 18 and 40 has had negative Pap smears for three consecutive years, the test may be performed less frequently at the discretion of her doctor. Starting at 40, she should have a Pap smear annually.

Nutrition and Diet

One of the most important lifestyle choices that affects your health is what you eat. Indeed, there is substantial evidence that your choice of diet can influence your risk for five of the 10 leading causes of death in the United States, including coronary heart disease, stroke, diabetes, atherosclerosis and certain forms of cancer. And while health experts urge people to make healthier food choices to avoid these chronic illnesses, which are responsible for about 68 percent of all deaths in the United States, many individuals nevertheless maintain a diet that is far from optimal.

Even though many people know that it would be beneficial to cut down on dietary fat and cholesterol, watch their sodium intake, and eat more foods rich in complex carbohydrates and fiber, they are not always certain about how to apply these principles in their daily lives.

A Balanced Diet

Fortunately, developing healthy eating habits is actually quite simple to do. The object is to eat a balanced diet consisting of many different types of foods, which does not emphasize any one particular category.

Choosing from a wide variety of foods — including fruits, vegetables, whole grains, pasta, legumes, low-fat milk products, lean meats, poultry and fish — not only gives you a broad range of nutrients in your diet, but it also lessens the chance that you will consume dangerous amounts of toxic substances and chemicals found in some foods.

Each type of food makes a slightly different nutritional contribution to your diet. In addition to eating familiar favorites, it is best to broaden your palate and try some unfamiliar foods as well, since this gives you the opportunity to enjoy new varieties and try exotic tastes. A healthy diet, after all, need not confine you to a lifetime of eating foods that are bland or unappealing.

Moderation is another important component of a healthy diet. A moderate eating plan involves alternating substitutions — for example, if you eat a fat-laden morning meal, select low-fat foods for the remainder of that day. It is unlikely that most people are going to abandon steak and french fries for tofu and alfalfa sprouts. But there is no reason why you need to give up all your favorite foods. Although eating steak every night is not recommended, there is nothing wrong with an occasional steak dinner.

Carbohydrates for Energy

Overall, no more than 30 percent of your calories should come from fat. Of the remainder, about 15 percent should come from protein, and by far the largest portion — at least 55 percent of your caloric intake — should come from carbohydrates, which are divided into two general types: simple and complex.

Simple carbohydrates are sugars, including glucose and fructose from fruits and vegetables, lactose from milk, and sucrose from cane or beet sugar. Refined and processed foods such as candy, cookies, cake, jams and many soft drinks contain mostly sucrose. Although these processed foods are dense in calories, they offer little else in the way of nutrients.

However, many natural foods containing simple sugars, such as fruits and juices, are good sources of vital nutrients as well.

Complex carbohydrates, which are made up of long chains of simple sugars, are found in a wide variety of plant foods, including breads, pasta, rice, beans and other legumes, cereals, fruits, potatoes, corn and a variety of vegetables. Unlike many refined foods that are loaded with sucrose, foods high in complex carbohydrates tend to be rich in vitamins and minerals and are often good sources of protein as well. Fruits, vegetables, legumes, rice and pasta do not contain any cholesterol, and they are low in fat.

As an added benefit, fiber is present in many complex carbohydrates. Foods containing insoluble fiber, such as whole grains, dried beans and peas and most fruits and vegetables, have been found to prevent constipation and may protect against colon cancer. Studies also suggest that another type of soluble fiber may be effective in reducing both cholesterol and triglyceride levels in your blood. Citrus fruits, apples, barley, carrots, okra, dried beans and peas, and unrefined oats are especially good sources of soluble fiber in your diet. Most foods that are high in fiber contain varying proportions of both soluble and insoluble types, so it is not necessary to keep track of which high-fiber carbohydrate foods you consume.

Moreover, carbohydrates are your most efficient source of energy. They are transformed into blood sugar glucose, which serves as your basic fuel. Contrary to what most people believe, carbohydrates are not fattening as long as you limit yourself to mod-

Making Healthy Choices

◆ For the most nutrients, choose fresh vegetables; frozen varieties are second best. Vegetables that are green and yellow and small and dark generally have the most vitamins and flavor. Vegetables in season usually offer the greatest value and quality.

◆ When buying produce, shop at farm stands whenever possible. When purchasing produce from greengrocers and supermarkets, select unwrapped fruits and vegetables so that you can inspect each piece individually and avoid buying bruised, wilted or damaged items.

◆ It is usually best to buy fresh fruits when they are in season and beginning to ripen. They should smell slightly sweet, and their texture should be firm, not hard. Berries should be purchased when they are ripe enough to eat, but choose slightly green bananas. Grapefruit should feel smooth and dense, and oranges should be firm and heavy.

◆ Buy beans in stores that have a high turnover of merchandise. Beans should be free of mold, dirt and debris, and their color should be bright. Choose beans of the same size and color. Pinhole marks and cracks in beans may indicate insect damage.

◆ When purchasing fish, be sure that it is fresh. Whole fish should have bright, bulging eyes, red gills, tight scales and firm flesh that springs back when it is touched. Fish should be virtually odorless, never "fishy."

◆ Buy the most lean grade of meat available. The U.S. Department of Agriculture grades meat by marbling and color, which indicates flavor and tenderness. Beef is graded prime, choice and good. The higher-priced prime and choice cuts have a greater fat content than good. Beef marked lean is usually graded as good. Among the most lean types of beef are top round, shoulder, eye round, top sirloin, flank and extra-lean ground.

◆ Chicken is classified as roaster, broiler, fryer or stewing hen. The most tender and lowest in fat is the small young roaster. It is generally best to buy fresh, not frozen, poultry.

erate amounts and do not smother them in rich sauces. Gram for gram, carbohydrates have the same number of calories as pure protein and less than half the calories of fat.

It is easy to get confused when confronted with a bewildering array of food choices. For guidance, just keep in mind the following basic rules of good nutrition:
- Get more than half of your daily calories from carbohydrates, concentrating on foods such as rice, potatoes and pasta.
- Eat plenty of fiber-rich foods, such as vegetables, whole grains and fruits, including the skins.
- Consume a relatively small amount of fat, especially the saturated

fats found in butter, fatty meats and tropical oils.
- Avoid too much sodium, sugar and cholesterol. If you drink alcohol, drink it in moderation.
- Avoid processed foods as much as possible. Processing generally removes fiber and nutrients while it adds unhealthy sodium and fats.

For tips on how to reduce your intake of fats, see pages 80-81; to cut down on cholesterol, see pages 64-65; to decrease alcohol consumption, see pages 52-53; to increase fiber intake, see pages 82-83. For information on how to order healthy foods in restaurants, see pages 76-77. See the box (above) for tips on selecting nutritious foods.

Over-the-Counter Drugs

By virtue of medicines that can be obtained without a prescription, people can treat themselves for numerous ailments that include headaches, hay fever, colds, cuts, constipation, sleeplessness, indigestion and other afflictions. Over-the-counter drugs are sufficiently potent to relieve symptoms and even cure and prevent certain illnesses and diseases.

According to the Federal Food, Drug, and Cosmetic Act, nonprescription drugs are safe without the supervision of a physician; they are not addictive if used correctly; and they must have clear warnings and instructions printed on the labels for consumer use and protection. Any over-the-counter drug can be dangerous, however, if taken in excess, by children, the elderly or pregnant women, or in combination with other types of drugs.

According to the law, nonprescription medications are not intended as treatment for serious problems, and they must be safe for general use without medical supervision. Today there are over 300,000 nonprescription drugs available in the United States. Researchers estimate that 60 percent of the medications in the average medicine cabinet are over-the-counter drugs.

A survey has suggested that people treat themselves with nonprescription drugs four times as often as they seek the care of a physician. And the growing trend is to make many previously designated prescription drugs, such as antihistamines, hydrocortisone ointments and fluoride rinses, directly available to consumers while providing sufficient directions and warnings approved by the FDA as well.

The Wide Choice Available

While pharmacists and doctors can offer help in choosing the most effective medication for a particular condition, many people rely on product labels and advertising when selecting over-the-counter drugs. The wide assortment and competing claims of nonprescription medications, however, can easily confuse people.

Simply finding a remedy for a sore throat may be a bewildering experience: Manufacturers offer mouthwashes, lozenges, sprays, drops, powders and chewing gums. These items include a variety of medications that function in different ways. For instance, those that include astringents reduce throat irritation by removing or by binding the protein elements from the mucosal cell surfaces; decongestants relieve congestion by shrinking the swollen tissue of the mucous membranes; and anesthetics and analgesics alleviate discomfort by decreasing overall sensitivity.

The Right Selection

Each product contains at least one FDA-approved active ingredient. For people familiar with the different types of medications, but unfamiliar with ingredients, selecting the most effective over-the-counter remedy for a particular condition may present a difficult task. Fortunately, because of FDA requirements, the product information on over-the-counter drug labels presents you with enough information to make an informed choice, as long as you carefully read the pro-

duct warnings, storage information, expiration date and directions.

Reading the labels carefully can also protect your health. While most items in over-the-counter drugs are generally considered safe, they can have side effects and produce adverse reactions when combined with other medications. Individuals who are taking prescription drugs, pregnant women, those buying over-the-counter remedies for children or the elderly and people with chronic medical conditions, such as hypertension or diabetes, should check with their doctors before taking any drugs. Those with dietary restrictions should also read labels with extra care because ingredients such as sodium, sugar and caffeine are included in many products. In addition, some medications should never be taken in conjunction with alcohol, since they may produce drowsiness, affect coordination and result in other unwanted side effects.

When buying over-the-counter drugs, be sure that the packages are sealed. Medicines that have been tampered with may cause serious harm or death. To discourage this, manufacturers now use safety seals, stickers and wrappings to guarantee tamper-proof drugs. Never purchase a product that appears tampered with or suspicious in any way.

Most individuals buy nonprescription medication for pain relief. Three of the most frequently used over-the-counter drugs for the alleviation of pain are aspirin, acetaminophen and ibuprofen. Unfortunately, many people use pain relievers interchangeably, without understanding their specific functions and properties. The chart (*opposite*) offers a guide to over-the-counter pain relievers.

Comparing Pain Relievers

	ASPIRIN	**ACETAMINOPHEN**	**IBUPROFEN**
Effective against	Pain, inflammation, fever	Pain, fever	Pain, inflammation, fever
Use	Headaches, arthritis, sprains, rheumatism; during healing process, may relieve pain; may diminish risk of heart attack and most common type of stroke caused by clotting if taken every other day	Reduces pain and fever; can be used for conditions that involve bleeding; children under 16 can use for chicken pox and flu; aspirin substitute for those with asthma, ulcers or gout, and for people who have nausea and stomach pain from aspirin; can be used after oral surgery	Fever, arthritic inflammation, joint pain and stiffness, backaches, tension headaches, fever and aches of a cold; reduces clotting; excellent for menstrual cramps
Side effects	May irritate the stomach or cause bleeding, bloody stool or ringing in the ears; frequent users may experience ulcers or anemia; allergic reactions include itching, rashes, wheezing and hives; may aggravate asthma and cause asthma attacks; kidney and liver damage may occur if taken often with laxatives	Rarely causes skin rashes, painful urination, bloody or cloudy urine, jaundice, and unusual bruising and bleeding; large doses may cause liver damage and death	May cause gastrointestinal problems, visual disturbances, itching, rashes and dizziness; may interfere with use of diuretics and antihypertensive drugs; may increase effects of anticoagulants
Who should not use	People with ulcers, asthma, gout, stomach bleeding and allergies to aspirin; pregnant and nursing women; children under 16 with chicken pox or flu; people with liver or kidney disease and those who drink alcohol heavily; users of anticoagulants, antidiabetic or arthritis medication; people undergoing surgery	People with liver or kidney disease or infection; alcoholics	People with aspirin allergies or ulcers; users of diuretics and medication for high blood pressure; children under 12; pregnant and nursing women; alcoholics
Warnings	May slightly increase risk of hemorrhagic stroke if taken regularly; do not combine with acetaminophen, ibuprofen or nonsteroid anti-inflammatory medication	Do not combine with aspirin	Do not combine with aspirin

Pain Management

Unfortunately, everyone experiences some form of physical pain, and in a single year, almost half of all Americans require medical treatment for pain. Unpleasant as it is, however, in most cases, pain serves an important physiological purpose. Quite simply, acute, short-term pain, which comes on suddenly due to an injury or illness, is a warning that is transmitted by your nerves to your brain.

Although a nervous reflex makes you pull your hand away from a hot iron, the pain that follows serves as a warning not to touch the iron again. Similarly, pain in your Achilles tendons indicates that you have run too hard or long; you should rest for a while or risk injuring your tendons.

However, pain messages can go awry, lasting far longer than necessary to serve as a warning. Such long-lasting pain without a purpose is called chronic, and it afflicts about 10 million Americans. Back pain, for instance, that continues long after a strained back should be healed, can be chronic. The reasons for it can be emotional, or it can result from symptoms of diseases such as arthritis or cancer. Regardless of its cause, chronic pain can be debilitating, affecting every aspect of a person's life.

Whether acute or chronic, pain is subjective: How it is experienced is difficult to quantify, since it varies with the person and the circumstance. Studies have shown that your pain threshold — the degree of pain needed for you to perceive or react to it — can be raised by as much as 45 percent when you are distracted. It can also be raised by such techniques as hypnosis or meditation. For example, many people cannot remember how they got certain bruises, probably because they were preoccupied when they bumped themselves. In

contrast, they are more likely to focus on pain if they are anxious or tired.

The variability of pain can make its treatment problematic, although acute pain can usually be treated successfully with drugs. Some of these pain relievers work locally by blocking the sensation of pain at the site. These include over-the-counter medications like aspirin, ibuprofen and acetaminophen as well as some prescription drugs.

Narcotics, such as morphine and codeine, work systemically to alter the perception of pain sent to your brain. Studies have shown that in one-third of pain sufferers, a placebo will also lessen pain. In one study, patients who had pain resulting from tooth extractions reported experiencing greater relief if placebos were administered to them by physicians instead of nurses or hospital technicians. Experts think this is because expectations of relief cause your body to release self-manufactured painkillers called endorphins. The illustration (*opposite*) shows how pain travels and methods for intercepting its path.

Chronic pain can be much more difficult to control. Because it often has an emotional component, or is exacerbated by anxiety or depression, many doctors used to think it was imagined by the patient, and either ignored it or provided potentially addictive pain-killing drugs to treat it.

More recent research has showed that all pain is real, even if it has an emotional root. For example, abdominal cramps due to anxiety are still real. In fact, some experts believe that chronic pain is a type of disease in itself, and needs to be treated separately from other medical problems. This has led to a proliferation of pain centers around the

Pain

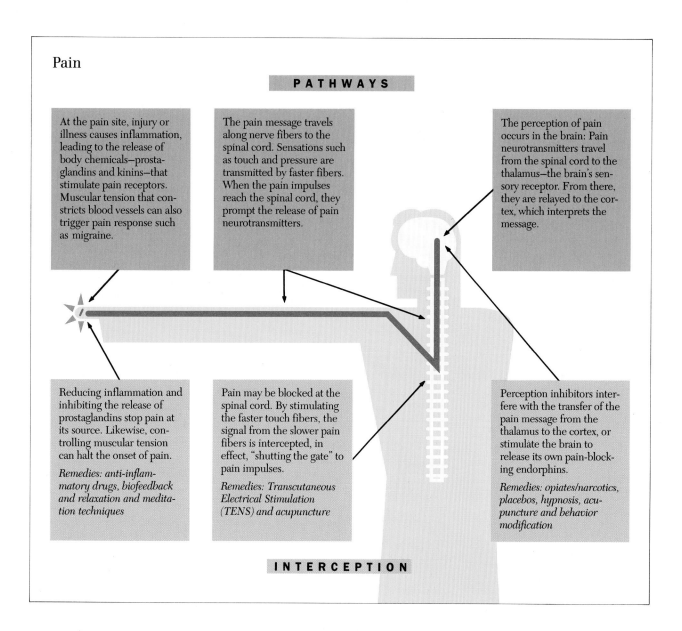

PATHWAYS

At the pain site, injury or illness causes inflammation, leading to the release of body chemicals—prostaglandins and kinins—that stimulate pain receptors. Muscular tension that constricts blood vessels can also trigger pain response such as migraine.

The pain message travels along nerve fibers to the spinal cord. Sensations such as touch and pressure are transmitted by faster fibers. When the pain impulses reach the spinal cord, they prompt the release of pain neurotransmitters.

The perception of pain occurs in the brain: Pain neurotransmitters travel from the spinal cord to the thalamus—the brain's sensory receptor. From there, they are relayed to the cortex, which interprets the message.

Reducing inflammation and inhibiting the release of prostaglandins stop pain at its source. Likewise, controlling muscular tension can halt the onset of pain.

Remedies: anti-inflammatory drugs, biofeedback and relaxation and meditation techniques

Pain may be blocked at the spinal cord. By stimulating the faster touch fibers, the signal from the slower pain fibers is intercepted, in effect, "shutting the gate" to pain impulses.

Remedies: Transcutaneous Electrical Stimulation (TENS) and acupuncture

Perception inhibitors interfere with the transfer of the pain message from the thalamus to the cortex, or stimulate the brain to release its own pain-blocking endorphins.

Remedies: opiates/narcotics, placebos, hypnosis, acupuncture and behavior modification

INTERCEPTION

country that are dedicated solely to the chronic-pain sufferer.

Pain centers are staffed by medical experts — including neurologists, orthopedists, psychotherapists and physical therapists. Pain specialists encourage chronic-pain patients to control their pain with various techniques. Sufferers can use behavior modification to sever the emotional aspect of pain, biofeedback to relax pain-related bodily responses and hypnosis to distract themselves from the pain. Physical stimulation of trigger points — nerve "hot spots" that, when activated, can block pain — also offer a drug-free way of coping. Both acupuncture, which is done with fine needles, and TENS — transcutaneous electrical nerve stimulation — which uses a device that can stimulate trigger points, can be effective for pain relief.

Any acute pain that is not relieved by an analgesic or worsens over a short period of time should send you to a physician for evaluation. If you suffer from chronic pain, you might want to consider a pain center; ask your doctor for a referral.

Pregnancy

Every aspect of your health takes on new meaning when you become pregnant, because taking care of your body will directly affect the health of your unborn child. If you are an expectant mother, or plan to become pregnant, you are certainly concerned with what is best for your baby, so you will need to evaluate your diet, exercise, work and lifestyle. In fact, pregnancy offers you an opportunity to make permanent improvements in these areas that will not only help to ensure a healthy baby, but can set the guidelines for healthy living.

While general issues of health, safety and nutrition apply to all pregnancies, each individual case differs, and it is of paramount importance that your condition be evaluated and monitored by your physician. Prenatal care should start as soon as you become pregnant, and any particular concerns that you have should be addressed to your doctor.

Nutritional Concerns

Because of the increased weight and energy demands associated with pregnancy, the most obvious areas you will need to measure and probably modify are nutrition and exercise. The demands of pregnancy will require, on average, 300 additional calories daily, often paired with a vitamin and/or iron supplement. Too many women increase their intake of fatty or sugary foods, instead of eating healthful ones, such as those shown in the chart *(right)*. Pregnancy is not an excuse for a binge; this leads to excess weight gain, which can complicate delivery and impede postpartum weight loss.

Pregnancy and Exercise

Pregnancy can also prompt positive changes in exercise habits — in fact, if you do not already exercise, pregnancy is a good time to begin. As recently as 20 years ago, doctors cautioned their patients to do only very mild exercise during pregnancy, but recent studies show that moderate exercise actually helps prevent such pregnancy-related complaints as back strain, varicose veins, hemorrhoids and constipation. Exercise also increases energy and improves your body image, and may even make labor and delivery easier.

The exercise you should perform depends on how fit you are and how you feel during pregnancy, and your needs may change month by month. The American College of Obstetricians and Gynecologists recommends that you target the same three fitness areas as nonpregnant women: aerobic endurance, muscular strength and flexibility. If you feel comfortable and your physician allows it, you can continue most forms of exercise right into your ninth month. However, you may have to make some modifications to compensate for your increasing weight, looser joints and impaired coordination. You may also want to perform exercises designed to meet your body's changing demands.

Averting Risks

Fortunately, averting the major risks to your unborn baby is within your control. Studies have shown that the three most dangerous toxins to your fetus are cigarettes, drugs and alcohol. All three can impair fetal development in different ways and should be avoided entirely.

The major danger of smoking is that cigarette smoke interferes with the flow of nutrition to your baby, and so can retard both its mental and physical growth, or even lead to miscarriage. Smokers generally have smaller babies than nonsmokers and studies have shown that, at age 11, children born to smokers are still shorter and have lower IQ scores than babies born to nonsmokers. While stopping smoking before pregnancy is best for both you and your baby, experts still strongly encourage quitting even if you are already pregnant.

Alcohol intake by pregnant women increases their risks of both miscarriage and low birth weight, and it is also a major cause of mental retardation. Heavy drinking can lead to a constellation of serious birth defects termed fetal alcohol syndrome. However, some studies have linked moderate drinking — even drinking during the very first weeks of pregnancy — with impaired growth and learning later in childhood. A fetus is exposed to the same level of alcohol as its mother when she drinks, but its liver cannot break it down.

Babies born to women who use illegal drugs can have life-threatening problems. However, most medications — both prescription and over-the-counter drugs — cross your placenta, which provides nourishment and oxygen to your fetus, and increase the chance of problems. You should consult your doctor before taking any medication, including aspirin and cough syrup, or if you have any medical condition that requires regular drug use.

The Healthy Pregnancy Diet

Adequate nutrition during pregnancy is essential for the health of both you and your baby. Ideally, you will gain 25 to 30 pounds; you should consume an additional 300 calories daily. (If you are a pregnant teenager, you will need even more additional calories; consult your doctor.) You should meet these caloric requirements with a nutritious diet based on the food groups and portions shown here.

FRUIT

4 servings per day
(one high in vitamin C)

1 serving fresh fruit (citrus fruits are high in vitamin C)

½ cup unsweetened frozen or canned fruit

4 oz fruit juice

VEGETABLES

3 or more servings per day
(one high in vitamin A)

1 cup raw vegetable (carrots and dark-green leafy vegetables are high in vitamin A)

½ cup cooked vegetable

4-6 oz vegetable juice

DAIRY PRODUCTS

4 servings per day

8 oz milk (whole, low-fat, skim or buttermilk)

8 oz plain yogurt

1½ oz hard cheese

1⅓ cups cottage cheese

BREADS AND CEREALS

10 servings per day
(at least 5 whole grain)

1 slice whole-grain bread

1 small muffin, roll or biscuit

½ cup cooked cereal, rice or pasta

¾ cup dry cereal

4-5 crackers

PROTEIN

5 servings per day
(animal and/or vegetable)

2 oz fish, poultry or lean meat

2 large eggs (limit 4 per week)

1 cup cooked legumes (beans, peas or lentils)

3-4 Tbsp peanut butter

6 oz tofu

POLYUNSATURATED FATS

6 servings per day

1 tsp oil, margarine or mayonnaise

2 tsp salad dressing

6 walnuts

10 almonds

Safe Sex

Everyone who is sexually active risks exposure to sexually transmitted diseases (STDs). Researchers have estimated that there are more than 50 of these diseases and syndromes, and the United States Public Health Service has reported that STDs, excluding AIDS, are responsible for an estimated 13 million cases and 7,000 deaths every year.

Exposure to STDs nearly always results from intimate contact with someone who is infected. When contact occurs, the organisms usually enter through the mucous membranes of your genitals, mouth or anus. Some STDs — such as AIDS, syphilis and herpes — can be spread without sexual contact. Other diseases only become STDs when their mode of transmission is sexual contact. Molluscum contagiosum, for instance, a viral skin infection, most frequently affects children who play together, but it can also infect adults through sexual contact. Catching STDs from objects such as toilet seats is almost impossible.

Most sexually transmitted diseases can be cured or at least controlled when detected and treated early. In later stages, when there has been organ damage, treatment is often more complicated. The consequences of untreated STDs can include blindness, brain damage, pelvic inflammatory disease, paralysis and death.

An obstacle in the treatment of STDs is the fact that many infected individuals are unaware of their condition and do not seek medical care. Chlamydia, for instance, which often has mild symptoms or none at all, is spreading — approximately 5 million new cases annually. Untreated chlamydia is a major cause of pelvic inflammatory disease and infertility in women.

STD Prevention

Abstention from sex is the only absolutely sure way to remain free of any disease that is acquired sexually. Monogamous couples also have little to fear. Those who are sexually active outside a monogamous relationship, however, should protect themselves from STDs by using barrier methods of birth control. Latex condoms and diaphragms used with spermicides are the most effective methods of protection. Used with a condom, nonoxydol-9, an ingredient in contraceptive jellies, creams and foams, is especially effective. Through a detergent action, nonoxydol-9 kills the AIDS virus and organisms that cause gonorrhea, syphilis, chlamydia, genital herpes and hepatitis B.

Unfortunately, no method is completely effective against all venereal diseases, and there are no vaccines available for any of them. Therefore, your first line of defense is knowing your sexual partners. If you have any doubt, you should use condoms to minimize any risk.

Protection from AIDS

AIDS — Acquired Immune Deficiency Syndrome — is caused by Human Immunodeficiency Virus (HIV). It is mainly spread through an exchange of semen or blood. It can also be spread through the use of unsterilized needles shared by drug addicts or by receiving contaminated blood transfusions. Once infected, most individuals remain asymptomatic for several years. However, 20 to 30 percent of infected individuals show symptoms of AIDS within five years, when HIV attacks the immune system and renders it incapable of fighting infection.

Although HIV infection can be deduced by finding the antibodies to the virus in blood tests, the antibodies may not appear for as long as three years after exposure. It is impossible to calculate how many people will become ill, since there is no way of knowing if all persons exposed to HIV will necessarily develop AIDS. The Centers for Disease Control estimates that there are one to 1.5 million Americans infected with HIV; it also predicts that 65,000 persons will die of AIDS in 1992.

Anyone who suspects that he or she has been exposed to the AIDS virus should immediately get tested. While there are currently no cures for AIDS, there are medications which inhibit viral replication.

If You Are Infected

Common symptoms of many STDs, except AIDS, include pain or a burning sensation when you urinate, discharge from your genitals, rashes, lesions, or itching or discomfort on or around your genitals. Many STDs, however, mimic the symptoms of other diseases and some may have no symptoms at all. If you suspect that you or your partner has been exposed to a sexually transmitted disease, consult your physician.

If you receive a positive test result for any STD, it is essential that you inform anyone with whom you have had sexual contact. Treatment for most STDs is quick and effective.

Sexually Transmitted Diseases

DISEASE	SYMPTOMS	HEALTH EFFECTS	TREATMENT
AIDS *Acquired Immune Deficiency Syndrome (HIV: Human Immuno-deficiency Virus)*	Persistent dry cough, swollen lymph nodes, skin lesions, fatigue, fever, night sweats, loss of appetite, weight loss, thrush, chronic diarrhea, increased susceptibility to infections, difficulty breathing. HIV-infected people may not show symptoms for years; they also may never develop AIDS.	Nearly always fatal. Virus disrupts immune defenses, making the person susceptible to infections and cancers. Kaposi's sarcoma, lymphoma and/or Pneumocystis carinii pneumonia often develop. Infection of brain cells can cause partial paralysis, loss of coordination or mental disorders.	Azidothymidine, or AZT, slows the virus. Other medications may also be beneficial.
Chlamydia *(Chlamydia trachomatis bacteria)*	Vaginal or penile discharge and urinary discomfort 10 days to several months after exposure; often extremely mild and ignored. Many people are asymptomatic.	Sterility, infertility, pelvic inflammatory disease, miscarriage, ectopic pregnancy, premature delivery and postpartum infection. The disease can be passed to newborns during delivery.	Antibiotics
Genital Herpes *(Herpes simplex virus)*	Itching or tingling in genital area and pain in the testicles two to 21 days after exposure. Blisters burst quickly and become painful sores. Symptoms usually stop within two weeks but often recur.	Increases risk of miscarriage, premature delivery and cervical cancer. Sores may infect infant during vaginal delivery, causing brain damage, blindness or death. Open sores may allow AIDS virus infection.	Acyclovir, xylocaine cream or ethyl chloride may reduce severity and frequency of sores.
Genital Warts *(Human Papilloma virus)*	Warts appear three weeks to three months after exposure. Because they may be hidden in the vagina, they are often undetected by women; extremely contagious.	Often more annoying than dangerous; may increase risk of developing cervical cancer and may increase the chance of contracting the AIDS virus, if exposed.	Chemical, dry ice or liquid nitrogen; may require cauterization or surgery.
Gonorrhea *(Gonococcus bacteria)*	Vaginal or penile discharge and painful urination occur two to 21 days after exposure. About 60 percent of women and some men have very mild symptoms or none at all. Can be mistaken for other conditions, such as a bladder infection.	May cause pelvic inflammatory disease in women; arthritis, meningitis and abscesses in men. Pregnant women can pass it on to newborns during delivery. May increase risk of contracting AIDS, if exposed.	Antibiotics
Syphilis *(Spirochete bacteria)*	Painless chancre, or sore, usually appears nine to 90 days after exposure. Most women and some men are unaware of infection. Chancre may disappear but swollen lymph glands in genital area, fever, mouth sores, sore throat, joint aches, hair loss and rashes can occur up to six months later.	Can affect any organ, causing paralysis, heart disease, blindness or insanity. Infection in women not treated within first four months of pregnancy can cause stillbirth, infant deformities or the disease. Open sores may allow AIDS virus infection, if exposed.	Penicillin, tetracycline

Sexuality

Beginning at conception and lasting until death, sexuality is an integral part of your personality. Feelings of masculinity or femininity, your gender roles in society, and sex drive are all aspects of your sexuality, just as lovemaking is. So powerful and compelling are these feelings that they influence your life from career to lifestyle to leisure activities.

At conception, a sperm cell fertilizes an egg cell, each of which contains 23 chromosomes bearing a set of genetic instructions. When combined, the 23 pairs of chromosomes provide the blueprint by which the fertilized egg will grow into a fetus and then become a child. One chromosome in each sperm carries the sex-determining factor — either an X or a Y. The egg always has an X chromosome, and if it is fertilized by an X sperm also, the XX fetus will be a girl; if the sperm has a Y chromosome, the XY fetus will be a boy.

Although sex is determined at conception, gender identity — your sense of maleness or femaleness — is programmed into the hypothalamus in your brain six to 12 weeks after conception. This is a critical period of development, since it prepares you for later sexual behavior.

By the age of three, most children already have a strong and secure sense of gender. This early awareness of sexuality results in significant behavioral differences between young girls and boys. In a study of 33 three-year-old children, each child sat in a chair with his or her back to a table. A toy was placed on the table and each child was told not to peek. Within five minutes after being left alone, only four children had not peeked. When the study conductor returned and asked if the children had peeked, 11 of them — nine boys — said they had, while another 11 — eight girls — said they had not. While the girls were no more likely to peek than the boys, they were far more likely to deny doing so, possibly because girls are more interested in social approval or feel more shame after committing an offense.

Puberty

During puberty, both males and females develop their secondary sexual characteristics — signs of sexual maturity. Their sex drives increase, and they become capable of reproduction. Hormones released from the hypothalamus begin this process. In males, the results include genital development, deepening of their voices, growth of body hair and muscle enlargement. In females, the hypothalamus controls the menstrual cycles, which begin at about age 13 and continue for about 35 years. The cycles are generally between 20 and 45 days long, and are normally interrupted only by pregnancy.

Sexual Behavior

The changes brought on by puberty prepare your mind and body for sex. Sexual behavior can be divided into three stages: Proceptive, acceptive and conceptive. The proceptive stage consists of attraction and courtship. It is experienced as sexual desire or interest, resulting in a range of behavior from a single sexual encounter to an ongoing sexual relationship such as marriage.

The acceptive stage begins with excitement and erection in males, and swelling and lubrication of the genital tissues in females. Excitement culminates in orgasm, which is a climactic feeling of sexual pleasure and release of tension, accompanied by generalized muscular contractions and pelvic thrusts. In males, orgasm includes ejaculation of semen. The acceptive phase concludes with generalized muscular relaxation.

The final stage of sexual behavior is the conceptive phase, which involves conception, pregnancy, childbirth and parenthood.

Sexual Problems

Problems can occur during any phase of sexual behavior. Impotence and frigidity are among the most common. Occasional impotence, the inability to maintain an erection, afflicts as many as 50 percent of men; 10 percent may be impotent all the time. About a third of all impotence cases have physical causes, such as diabetes, previous prostate or urological surgery, hormonal problems, alcoholism or the use of medications or drugs. Most cases, however, have a psychological root, such as anxiety, depression, negative self-image or marital problems. About 80 percent of all cases of impotence with a psychological origin can be overcome with therapy.

Frigidity is a label used for a wide range of sexual dysfunctions in women. Unfortunately, the term implies coldness. Frequently, a "frigid" woman may become sexually excited but unable to achieve orgasm. However, surveys indicate that only about 30 percent of women are able to

Older Can Be Better

Recent research has shown that many people enjoy active sex lives well into their old age. Indeed, according to a Duke University study, 80 percent of men in their late sixties are still interested in sex. At the age of 78 and beyond, one in four men continues to be sexually active. Women can also have active sex lives in their later years; decreased sexual activity among older women often results from lack of a partner rather than lack of interest.

◆ Do not assume that sexual problems are the inevitable results of aging. Counseling and sex therapy can often resolve even those problems that have persisted for years.

◆ Sex can improve for women after menopause, since they no longer have to be concerned with menstrual cycles and birth control.

◆ As they age, men often find that it takes them longer to achieve orgasm. Longer foreplay with less urgency about reaching climax can improve your feelings of intimacy with your spouse.

◆ Remember that not every sexual experience must end with an orgasm. Focusing sexual activity toward orgasm can cause anxiety and even result in impotence. Instead, agree with your spouse not to have orgasm during sex; this may relieve performance anxiety so that you can be more free to enjoy the sensuality of sex.

◆ Continue to practice good hygiene, regular exercise and proper nutrition to stay in the best-possible physical condition.

◆ Avoid big meals just before having sex, since they may produce distracting feelings of fullness and discomfort. Also, alcohol and cigarettes can suppress sexual functioning.

◆ If you are too tired for sex in the evening, try again at another time of day, such as in the morning when you are more relaxed and refreshed.

achieve orgasm during intercourse; up to two-thirds of females need direct stimulation of their clitoris for orgasm. As with male impotence, frigidity may also have organic or psychological causes.

One of the most common of all sexual problems is a condition known as Inhibited Sexual Desire, or ISD. This syndrome is often the result of stress due to depression, anger, anxiety, guilt or concern about self- or body image. If you suffer from ISD, you should consult a physician, since it may be the result of a medical condition. However, if it is caused by stress, you can often reduce it through stress management (see pages 122-123).

Exercise not only reduces anxiety and depression, it also improves your self-image and possibly your sex life. Physically fit individuals are more likely to feel good about their bodies and less ashamed about their appearance or inhibited sexually than people in poor physical condition. For information on how to begin an exercise program that will improve your fitness level, see pages 84-85.

Most healthy couples can enjoy sex well into their later years. For tips on keeping the flame alive, see the box *(above)*. For information on pregnancy, see pages 110-111. For tips on safe sex and how to avoid getting sexually transmitted diseases (STDs), turn to pages 112-113.

Sleep

The relationship between sleeping and health is still a mystery, since we do not know why sleep is necessary. However, researchers have discovered a great deal about what occurs during sleep, what disturbs it and how to improve your sleep habits.

Sleep appears to restore you physically. You alternate between periods of REM (rapid eye movement) sleep, during which you dream, and a deep-sleep phase that grows progressively deeper. Studies have revealed that during periods of deep sleep, your body releases most of its supply of growth hormone, which some scientists think is responsible for renewing worn-out tissues. Other studies link growth hormone to the formation of red blood cells. Male testosterone hormone secretion is much greater during sleep than it is in waking hours.

The most important benefit of sleep may be that it leaves you feeling refreshed mentally. A lack of sleep appears to affect your mind far more dramatically than your body. If you stay awake for 24 hours, you are likely to feel quite fatigued, your attention will wander, and you may experience mood shifts, headaches and blurred vision. How sleeplessness affects your mental ability depends on the amount of sleep deprivation and the task involved. According to one study, your creativity and ability to deal with new situations can diminish after you lose a night's sleep. However, sleep loss does not appear to compromise your ability to handle mechanical or logical tasks, using well-established skills.

The effect of sleep loss on your physical performance also depends on the complexity of the activity. In studies of subjects who stayed awake for 30 to 50 hours, researchers found little change in such indicators of exertion as heart rate and oxygen intake. On the other hand, physical activities that require a variety of skills, such as playing tennis, may be more difficult if you are deprived of sleep than repetitive activities such as cycling or running. Fortunately, you can make up for lost sleep very quickly. Studies of people deprived of sleep for days show that most of them can recover after only one long night's sleep.

It is a widely held belief that most people need eight hours of sleep every night to function at their best. However, experts emphasize that you have had a good night's sleep if you feel refreshed and alert the next day, which allows for wide variations in the amount of sleep required for that condition. Some people need ten hours; others require only five or six. Age is one of the most important factors governing sleep requirements. Infants may sleep 18 or more hours a day. By early adolescence, children have reached their adult sleeping patterns. The next noticeable shift occurs after age 60, when sleep for most people becomes increasingly fragmented. At that time, you tend to wake up more frequently and periods of deep, restful sleep grow shorter.

Younger people can also experience fragmented, interrupted sleep. In fact, about 15 to 20 percent of American adults have insomnia — a term that refers to having trouble falling asleep or continuing it. Insomnia has many causes: It can be temporary, as when you have jet lag or are anxious about a specific situation; or it can be chronic, in which case it may be caused by underlying medical or psychological conditions. In many cases, insomnia persists because of habits or patterns

Getting a Good Night's Sleep

If you have difficulty falling asleep, or if you do not wake up feeling refreshed and alert, the following suggestions should help make falling asleep less stressful and also improve the quality of your sleep:

◆ Relax an hour or so before going to bed. Listen to music, read or enjoy a warm — but not hot — bath. Do not take troubles or work to bed with you. If you want to exercise in the evening, finish up two hours before bedtime.

◆ Do not have coffee, tea or caffeinated colas within four hours of bedtime. Do not smoke; the nicotine in tobacco is a stimulant. And skip having a nightcap — it will disrupt your sleep.

◆ Keep your bedroom dark, quiet and at a comfortable temperature — for most people, 60 to 65 degrees is satisfactory. Do not overdress yourself for bed; it is better to have an extra blanket available that you can cover yourself with if you get cold.

◆ Try to go to bed at the same time each night, but only if you feel drowsy. If you cannot fall asleep in 15 or 20 minutes, leave your bedroom and return only when you are sleepy. No matter how poorly or how little you sleep, get up at the same time — and do not take naps during the day. Also, do not try to make up for lost sleep on weekends.

◆ Counting sheep—or performing some other simple, repetitive routine—can help you relax in bed. Or try progressive relaxation: Tense, then relax, each muscle group, starting at your toes and working up to your head.

◆ If you experience severe or chronic insomnia, you should see a doctor or go to a sleep-disorder clinic to see if you have an underlying medical condition.

that reinforce it, which include working in bed, attempting to sleep at erratic times and using sleeping pills, alcohol or other drugs.

Many people assume that prescription sleeping pills, which are among the most frequently used drugs in the United States, are adequate sleeping aids as long as they are not used to the point of dependency. In fact, both sleeping pills and alcohol ultimately interfere with natural sleeping patterns rather than aid them. Although sleeping pills may improve sleep temporarily, they eventually result in fragmented sleep, upsetting dreams and fatigue during the day. Moreover, when taken nightly, some sleeping pills may lose their effectiveness in less than a week. As with other habituating drugs, you can end up increasing

the dosage to obtain the same effect, which increases side effects and the risks of developing an addiction and having an overdose.

At most, you should use sleeping pills only occasionally, and never for more than three successive nights. If you are pregnant or take other medications, you should avoid sleeping pills completely. If you have any medical conditions, particularly liver or kidney problems, you should consult your doctor before taking sleeping pills. Never combine sleeping pills with alcohol.

A nightcap of alcohol by itself will not be a useful aid, either. Alcohol may help you fall asleep, but your sleep will probably be light and uneasy rather than restful. The advice in the box (*above*) should prove more effective at enhancing sleep.

Smoking

Cigarette smoking is the number-one public-health risk, primarily because it is directly linked with heart attack and lung cancer. Smoking is also associated with a wide variety of other illnesses and cancers, including those of the mouth, esophagus, breast, cervix, and bladder.

The list of diseases associated with cigarette smoking is growing all the time. It is abundantly clear that smoking is the single most preventable cause of death and disability in the United States. It is equally true that if you smoke, kicking the habit is the most healthful decision you will make in your lifetime.

Why People Smoke

Surveys show that most people who smoke would like to quit, yet most attempts to give up the habit have failed. Only about 20 percent of people manage to quit on their first attempt. Nicotine, which is the active ingredient in tobacco smoke, is an insidious drug because it does not produce dramatic evidence of intoxication — its addictive power is often underestimated.

While producing no obvious changes in personality or behavior, nicotine does cause marked alterations in your body chemistry, acting through specialized cell formations in your brain and muscles. Once inhaled, nicotine goes to your brain almost immediately, producing a mild state of euphoria, particularly when you smoke your first cigarette of the day.

Without being aware of it, most smokers carefully regulate their intake of nicotine in order to maintain steady levels of it in their blood; they take more or fewer puffs, they inhale more or less deeply, and they pace their cigarettes unconsciously. What appears to be casual or random behavior is, in fact, steered by nicotine addiction. Failure to maintain steady blood levels of nicotine can result in symptoms of withdrawal, including anxiety, nervousness, loss of concentration and headaches.

Smoking is not simply a matter of nicotine addiction, however. Typically, an adolescent starts smoking to gain peer approval or admiration, to express rebelliousness, or simply out of curiosity. Many people take up smoking because their role models do it. Cigarette advertisers shrewdly take advantage of this motivation by presenting male cigarette smokers as rugged individualists and female smokers as attractive, young, thin and liberated. Companies that sell cigarettes sponsor athletic events, associating tobacco products with athletic performance.

As people begin to smoke, many of them learn that just handling cigarettes can be a pleasurable activity, one that is associated with the enjoyment of mealtime, or the end of classes or work, or with the relief of stress and tension.

Learning to Quit

Although quitting smoking is difficult, 32 million Americans gave up the habit between 1964 and 1985. Nearly every method, no matter how odd it may seem, has worked for somebody. If you know former smokers, interview them. Find out which method worked for them, why they may have failed on their first attempts and how they finally kicked the habit.

About 95 percent of all American ex-smokers were able to give up smoking without formal treatment programs. Studies show that about 20 percent of all those who quit for at least a day are still nonsmokers after a year. About 60 percent of all those who try to quit on their own can succeed with repeated attempts. Remember that most people fail on their first few attempts; use your failures as learning experiences so that you can avoid making the same mistakes in the future.

Staying Off

Many smokers who manage to give up cigarettes for a few days remark on how easy it is to do it. The withdrawal symptoms can be mild and last only three days to two weeks, and the rewards of not smoking soon become apparent. Your senses of smell and taste become enhanced; some ex-smokers have remarked that these senses are suddenly improved.

In addition, your breathing will be easier and your stamina will likely increase. Within the first year of quitting, most ex-smokers feel that they have more control over their health and well-being, and are less anxious or prone to depression than they had been previously. Ex-smokers also report less frequent use of drugs and alcohol.

Most smokers fear a weight gain after stopping their tobacco habits. This is partly due to an increase in appetite, which includes more snacks and desserts as substitutes for cigarettes, and a slight decline in metabolism. To counter this tendency,

Kicking the Habit

Since the circumstances under which you give up cigarettes can determine your ability to keep away from them for that first crucial day or two, choosing the right time to quit can be almost as important as your decision to do it. Many people, for instance, decide to stop smoking on a Monday morning, only to find themselves lighting up again in the early afternoon. Instead, plan to stop on a Friday afternoon so that you have the entire weekend away from your usual daily hassles, which may lead you to smoke. Better yet, plan a camping trip or some other activity so that you are away from your usual environment and can resist the easy temptation of cigarettes. The following tips may also be useful:

◆ Quit "cold turkey." In one study, over 90 percent of successful ex-smokers were found to have quit by giving up cigarettes abruptly. Those who taper down slowly or chew nicotine-flavored gum maintain their nicotine habits at a lower intensity. While the damage to your health caused by cigarettes is related to the amount that you smoke, there is no safe level of smoking.

◆ Start an aerobic exercise program. Now that you have given up smoking, you will have the stamina for vigorous exercise. Experts note that performing a regular exercise program is one of the best predictors of stopping smoking for good. Follow the guidelines on pages 84-85. Soon you may be running up the same stairs that once made you gasp for air. In addition to all of its other benefits, aerobic exercise will also help to keep your weight down.

◆ If you have cravings for cigarettes, remember that they usually last only a few minutes at a time. Deep abdominal breathing and some of the relaxation techniques explained on pages 122-123 may help you get through these brief periods.

◆ Remember that for each pack of cigarettes you do not smoke, you will live an estimated 137 minutes longer than if you did smoke it; you will also collect $1.82 in pension funds that would have gone to someone else. Use that time and money to reward yourself for not smoking: Treat yourself to dinner or go to the movies. Persons who used self-rewards were shown in one study to be more successful at abstaining from cigarettes than those who did not reward themselves.

◆ If you would prefer to enlist yourself in a stop-smoking program, there are plenty of groups available. Your local library or chapter of the American Cancer Society can supply information. Look in the Yellow Pages under "Smoker's Information and Treatment Centers." Be sure to stick with established stop-smoking programs, since hypnosis, acupuncture, electric shock, and chemical and dietary programs have not been proven to be effective.

keep low-calorie foods on hand, such as raw vegetables, fruits and unbuttered popcorn. The fear of weight gain is so powerful among some smokers that it may prevent them from making serious attempts to quit. Keep in mind, however, that not everyone gains weight after quitting. To maintain a proper diet, see pages 104-105. For tips on losing weight, see 130-131.

Some experts believe that the toughest part of giving up cigarettes is not the initial withdrawal period, or even the first year or so after quitting. After a few years, the memory of all the negative aspects of smoking begins to fade; meanwhile, many individuals develop an over-confidence in their ability to control it. At some point, stress at work, family pressures, or some change in association with the availability of cigarettes, leads some people to begin smoking again, sometimes 10 or 20 years after they had quit. For tips on quitting and advice on remaining that way, see the box *(above)*.

Sports Injuries

In the last two decades, the number of participants in virtually all sports and exercise activities has increased tremendously, along with the proliferation of sports-medicine clinics. During a five-year period at a large sports-medicine clinic in San Francisco, it was determined that injuries from running were by far the most common, although dance and tennis injuries also accounted for a large proportion.

Perhaps no group of recreational athletes has been studied more than runners. In a survey of 2,500 randomly selected participants in a 6.2-mile run, it was found that more than one-third of them had experienced musculoskeletal injuries within a year of the race.

Despite the apparent prevalence of sports injuries, however, it has been noted that most of them are minor and require little or no treatment beyond rest. Fear of injury should never stop you from exercising. If you use proper equipment and do not overtrain, you will most likely avoid major mishaps. If, during the course of maintaining your physical health and vitality, you happen to suffer an occasional muscle strain, blister or bout of soreness, you may decide that it is a small price to pay for the many life-enhancing benefits of being active.

Most injuries can be divided into two general categories: acute and stress. Acute injuries occur suddenly, such as a bruise or sprained ankle. These are most likely to happen during team and contact sports like football and basketball. Stress injuries often develop over time, beginning as minor discomforts and then increasing in severity until they require treatment. Stress injuries occur most frequently during continuous activities such as running or cycling. (See the chart opposite.)

Of course, everyone who exercises or engages in sports should expect occasional minor aches and pains. Indeed, many athletes use their sense of discomfort as a gauge of their physical effort. Unfortunately, pain is not a reliable indicator of the extent of an injury, and it is sometimes easy to misinterpret. A minor muscle cramp, for instance, can be quite painful for a few minutes but have no lasting results. On the other hand, many people ignore the symptoms of a stress fracture because the pain — if it even causes pain at all — is relatively minor. The result can be a complete break in your bone.

For minor injuries with no obvious swelling, you can often recover simply by not exercising for a few days or by cutting back on the intensity and duration of your activity. For injuries with swelling and pain or a burning sensation, however, you should apply "RICE," which stands for rest, ice, compression and elevation. Stop exercising and do not do anything that causes pain. Apply ice as soon as possible to the injured area, which acts as a local anesthetic and reduces swelling.

For surface injuries, freeze water in Styrofoam or paper cups that you can use to rub the ice gently around the injured area. For deeper injuries, crush ice and wrap it in a towel before applying it to your body. Never apply ice for longer than 30 minutes at a time.

Apply compression whenever there is swelling and fluid accumulation. Wrap an elastic bandage snugly but not tightly around the

Injuries

	STRESS	ACUTE
Onset	Insidious: usually difficult to determine cause	Sudden: obvious cause
Cause	Repeated microtrauma, biomechanical imbalance; often occurs after increase in training intensity or frequency	Single traumatic experience
Activity	Do not overtrain; depending on the severity, cut back on activity or stop entirely until symptoms subside.	Begin gentle stretching exercises after swelling stops; wait until injury is 75 percent healed before resuming activity.
Treatment	R.I.C.E.* (Rest, Ice, Compression, Elevate); adhesive taping may relieve discomfort; if pain persists, consult a physician.	See a physician or sports-medicine professional if injury affects bones, joints or ligaments or if you have any doubts. R.I.C.E.* can be helpful in some cases, such as sprains and pulled muscles.
Prevention	Adopt a stretching and strengthening program. Set realistic goals and do not overtrain. Use proper equipment.	Participate in a stretching and strengthening program. Warm up before exercising. Wear safety equipment and play by the rules when participating in team sports. Do not exercise strenuously when overtired, weak or in pain.

*Never use ice if you have circulatory problems or if you are hypersensitive to cold.

injured area. To apply ice and compression at the same time, wrap the crushed ice in a towel under the elastic bandage. Injuries that result in swelling should also be elevated, particularly if it involves an extremity, such as an ankle sprain. Raising the injury will reduce the accumulation of fluids.

Do not hesitate to see a physician if you have any doubt about the extent or nature of your injury. Be particularly wary of joint injuries: You should always see a doctor if a joint injury restricts your movement. Also, be sure to consult a physician if the injury fails to heal or if infection develops and you have a fever or pus around the area.

Once the swelling has stopped, you can begin gentle stretching exercises. After the swelling disappears, begin exercising slowly and moderately. To avoid re-injury, stop exercising immediately whenever you feel pain.

Of course, you should always take prudent steps to avoid injury in the first place. Be sure to wear protective equipment. Cyclists, for instance, should not only ride a properly adjusted and well-maintained bicycle, but they should wear helmets in case of accidents, and cycling shoes and toe clips on the pedals to reduce strain on their ankles and knees. Cycling gloves and shorts can also aid in comfort and minimize chafing. Runners and fitness walkers should wear proper shoes. For tips on choosing the right athletic shoes for you, see pages 90-91.

Stress Management

Many people feel that they are adrift in a sea of stress — helplessly buffeted by job problems, commuting hassles, financial pressures and troubles at home. Yet, it is unlikely that modern man suffers from the ill effects of stress any more than his prehistoric predecessors. The only difference may be that modern man has studied stress extensively: More than 150,000 studies and articles have been devoted to the subject, as well as numerous books.

Prior to the 1980s, most stress research concentrated on its harmful effects. People were warned to avoid stress or suffer the consequences. However, stress can mean different things to various people: One person can perceive an impending deadline as highly stressful and literally become sick; another may accept the deadline as a challenge and rise to the occasion, producing exceptionally imaginative and perceptive work. In the last ten years, more researchers have focused on how stress can be beneficial.

Using Stress Positively

One line of investigation has tracked how athletes can use their perceived stress, or arousal, to enhance their performance. One Soviet psychologist has determined that there is a zone of optimal functioning. If your arousal level is below your zone of optimal functioning, you may feel bored, listless or unmotivated, and your performance will show it.

On the other hand, if your arousal level is above your optimal zone, you will be too nervous or you will con-

centrate too much on inconsequential details, and your performance will be equally poor.

Arousal levels can be measured by analyzing stress hormones in your blood and measuring your heart rate and blood pressure. Athletes who perceive they have reached their optimal zones of arousal describe themselves as being "psyched up." The Soviets determined that highly skilled athletes generally need elevated levels of arousal to do their best performance.

In the United States, important research into the positive aspects of stress has centered on business executives. One recent study investigated Illinois Bell executives who thrived during the breakup of the corporation *(see pages 38-39)*. It was discovered that executives who warded off the ill effects of stress most effectively viewed the corporate upheaval as a challenge. These executives, who the researchers described as "hardy," welcomed the changes because they presented new opportunities. Other executives, however, felt threatened by the breakup; these people felt alienated and powerless. Feeling the typical effects of stress, the threatened individuals took sick days nearly twice as often as the "hardy" executives.

Dealing with Confrontations

Psychologists have shown that people tend to cope with stressful situations at work in either resentful or reflective manners. Researchers subdivide the resentful people into two categories of groups: "anger-in" and "anger-out."

In one study, subjects were asked how they would respond if their bosses suddenly reprimanded them for no reason. Anger-in respondents said they would walk away from the situation and try to ignore it; anger-out respondents said they would report the boss to a superior or to the union. Anger-In respondents, the researchers found, had elevated blood pressures. This may correlate to their tendencies not to confront and resolve problems, harboring lingering feelings of resentment. Surprisingly, anger-out copers tended to have even higher blood pressure readings, perhaps because their methods of confrontation often lead to ongoing conflicts with authorities.

Those with the lowest blood pressures were the reflective copers or those who said they would try to reason with their bosses at the time of the reprimands or wait until they had cooled down before trying to respond. The researchers believed that their subjects dealt with a wide variety of stressful situations, not just with unreasonable bosses, in similar fashions. Reflective copers focus on problems and try to solve them, instead of retaliating or harboring angry feelings.

Researchers believe that many people respond to stressful home situations in much the same way they deal with difficult work circumstances. Most professionals agree that regardless of people's methods of dealing with stress, it is best to communicate openly with family and friends who can offer support and understanding. Often, individuals try to isolate their families from the stresses of their jobs. When events are not going well at work, for instance, many people will not tell

Learning to Relax

While there are a wide variety of techniques that can help you reduce stress and increase your level of relaxation, all of them have one aspect in common — deep breathing, which has been proven to lower your heart rate. In practicing any of the techniques below, inhale and exhale deeply, focusing your attention on the way your body feels when you do it. When you inhale, fill your lungs so that your abdomen protrudes, then slowly release the air. Deep breathing can increase the quantity of air taken into your lungs by approximately 15 percent, raising the potential for a more significant exchange of oxygen and carbon dioxide. Even a single deep breath has been shown to lower your heart rate. Not every relaxation technique will work well for everyone. Meditation, for instance, can actually increase anxiety in some people; for them, some other method may be more useful. Here are some of the most popular relaxation techniques.

◆ **Biofeedback.** Although most biofeedback machines are expensive laboratory devices, some inexpensive home models are available. The machines measure your muscle tension, skin conductivity or temperature or blood pressure. The measurements are then displayed continuously on a monitor, either as numbers or as high- or low-pitched sounds. By using the display or sounds as a guide, many people can consciously lower their readings.

◆ **Progressive relaxation.** Lie down in a quiet room and breathe deeply. Tense the muscles around your eyes as tightly as you can for five seconds, then relax them. Tense your jaw muscles, then relax them. Work your way down your body, tensing and relaxing each muscle or muscle group, until you perform the procedure with your toes.

◆ **Transcendental meditation.** This involves using a special word, sound or phrase (a mantra) that you choose or receive from an instructor. You then sit in a comfortable position and repeat this mantra over and over again to displace all distracting thoughts and so attain a calm level of consciousness. Practice this procedure for 20 minutes every morning and evening.

◆ **Visualization.** Also known as imaging and mental rehearsal, visualization can help reduce anxiety and develop your capacity for experiencing a state of relaxed alertness. To be most effective, visualization should be performed when you are completely at ease. Take several deep breaths and imagine yourself in a relaxing scene, such as a deserted beach or a country field. Imagine the sights, sounds and smells in as precise detail as possible.

◆ **Yoga.** Instructors in Hatha Yoga teach their pupils various exercises to stretch and relax their muscles, and certain postures and breathing techniques to achieve voluntary control of their respiration. The lotus position — sitting with your legs crossed and your feet on your thighs — keeps your spine erect and allows your lungs to inhale and exhale easily. Studies have shown that Yoga practitioners are able to decrease their heart rate, respiration, and alpha-wave activity and achieve a deep relaxation of certain aspects of their autonomic nervous system without experiencing drowsiness or sleep.

---

their spouses. While the cause of stress can be concealed, the stress itself most often cannot, leading the spouse to believe something is wrong in the relationship. This frequently compounds the problem.

While there are inherent dangers in expressing too much anger and frustration, researchers point out that engaging in problem-focused coping — openly discussing problems as they arise with the objective of solving them — is often the best chance of dealing successfully with all types of stress.

In addition to utilizing constructive coping behaviors, many people can lower their perceptions of stress by engaging regularly in aerobic exercise, which is associated with a sense of well-being and a reduction of anxiety and depression. Also, regular aerobic exercise reduces the incidence of many stress-related illnesses, including hypertension, coronary artery disease and stroke. See pages 84-85 for tips on starting an exercise program. The box (above) lists several effective techniques to reduce stress.

Sun Safety

While most varieties of plants require exposure to sunlight for survival, people need it merely to maintain good health. The sun has many physical and psychological benefits. Its ultraviolet rays provide your daily requirement of vitamin D and prevent you from getting rickets. Moderate exposure to the sun is known to alleviate conditions such as acne, asthma and psoriasis, and recent studies indicate that it can also help prevent depression.

Too much sun can be harmful, however. Overexposure to sunlight is the major culprit in an estimated 500,000 cases of skin cancer in the United States annually. Sunlight also ages your skin prematurely and it can damage your eyes. Unfortunately, the harmful effects of the sun's rays are only likely to increase in the future. Because the earth's ozone layer — the atmospheric shield that filters the sun's rays — has been gradually dissipating during the past several years, many researchers believe that people have been and will continue to be overexposed to the sun's harmful ultraviolet light. Luckily, there are many ways to protect yourself.

Sunlight and Your Skin

The sun radiates many types of light: There is infrared light that you feel as heat, light that you are able to see, and invisible ultraviolet (UV) light. Two types of UV radiation affect your skin: UV-A rays tan your skin, while UV-B rays burn it. Both UV-A and UV-B rays damage the connective tissues and the blood vessels of your skin, thus promoting the aging

process. Infrared rays may also damage your skin, but this has not been proven as yet.

Excessive exposure to the sun may hasten the process that makes your skin sag. In addition, too much sun also thickens your skin, which accounts for the leathery appearance of many people who are exposed to sunlight constantly.

Your skin has its own sunscreen protection, which is called pigment. Generally, people with dark skin have more protection from the sun's damaging rays than fair-skinned individuals. However, pigment is not a perfect protection, since everyone can get sunburned no matter how dark his or her skin is. Similarly, dark-skinned people are also susceptible to premature aging of the skin and cancer, but light-skinned people burn most quickly and must protect themselves by using sunscreen and sun block. Even tanned skin needs some protection. You should apply a sunscreen whenever you plan to be in the sun for any length of time, even if you are naturally dark or you are already tanned. For tips on sunscreens, see the box (*opposite*).

Protecting Your Eyes

Your eyes need protection from the sun, too. Exposure to UV rays over the years can damage the lenses of your eyes, leading to potential cataracts, and UV rays have been implicated in damage to your corneas and retinas as well. Blue-violet light in wavelengths beyond UV may also damage your retinas. Of the million cataracts removed each year in the United States, it is estimated that up to 100,000 cases may be prevent-

ed with the use of better protection from the sun.

Do not assume that you are protecting your eyes just because you wear dark glasses. Sunglasses that do not have special UV block may, in fact, cause your eyes more harm, since they will make your pupils dilate, permitting more UV light to enter than if you wore no glasses at all.

Clear glass lenses alone naturally filter out the UV-B rays, but the harmful UV-A rays must be blocked with a special clear coating. Polycarbonate lenses, which now account for a high percentage of all spectacle lenses, block all UV radiation and blue-violet light without causing color distortion. These lenses can be obtained tinted, clear and in bifocal prescriptions.

When purchasing sunglasses, make sure that the lenses have been specially treated to protect against ultraviolet rays and blue light. Sunglass manufacturers, with approval from the Food and Drug Administration, voluntarily label nonprescription sunglasses in three classifications: cosmetic, general and special purpose. The cosmetic variety blocks at least 70 percent of UV-B rays and 20 percent of UV-A. General purpose sunglasses block 95 percent UV-B and at least 60 percent UV-A. Sunglasses classified as special purpose must block at least 99 percent UV-B and as well as 60 percent UV-A rays.

Benefits of Sunlight

While it is essential to guard against skin and eye damage in the sun, moderate exposure to sunlight can make you feel happier and healthier

Choosing Sunscreens

When spending time in the sun — walking, gardening, swimming or cycling — you can safeguard your skin by wearing protective clothing and using sunscreen that will help you avoid harm from dangerous ultraviolet rays. While sunscreens cannot protect you entirely, they can reduce the risk of sun damage if used with care. For optimal effectiveness, most screens should be applied 30 to 45 minutes before exposure; they must be reapplied generously and frequently. Keep in mind that the closer you are to the equator and the higher your altitude, the greater the intensity of the sun. Ultraviolet rays are also strongest between the hours of ten o'clock in the morning and three o'clock in the afternoon. Before choosing a sunscreen, you may find it helpful to understand a few of the elements that different products advertise. The sun's rays can be particularly intense in highly reflective environments, such as areas near water, snow or sand.

◆ Sun Protection Factor, or SPF, refers to the length of time you can remain in the sun without burning, as compared to the time you could stay in the sun without any sunscreen protection at all. For instance, if you have a fair complexion and would normally burn in 10 minutes, an SPF 8 sunscreen would allow you to stay in the sun for 80 minutes without burning. The American Cancer Society recommends people who spend long periods of time outdoors use an SPF of 15 or greater.

◆ SPFs with the same rating do not necessarily provide equal protection. The SPF number refers to how long you will be protected from the UV-B rays, which are primarily responsible for burning your skin. However, the UV-A rays are also dangerous; some sunscreens contain chemicals that guard you from the UV-A and UV-B rays, and others protect you only from the UV-B rays. When choosing a sunscreen, read the label carefully to be sure that the contents include at least two anti-ultraviolet ingredients to protect you from a range of light waves.

◆ Some sunscreens are advertised as waterproof and water resistant. The FDA requires that water-resistant screens must protect you for 40 minutes in the water at the SPF level on the label. Waterproof sunscreens must maintain their SPF levels for 80 minutes in the water. When using sun blocks or sunscreens, keep in mind that sweating can reduce their effectiveness; if you sweat profusely, use waterproof sunscreens.

◆ The American Academy of Dermatology has warned that some of the higher SPF formulas may cause skin irritation because their chemicals are so concentrated. If you reapply an SPF 8 or SPF 15 sunscreen at the proper intervals, you will have the same protection as with higher-rated sunscreens that need not be applied as frequently.

◆ Sun blocks — opaque creams or pastes containing zinc oxide or titanium dioxide — provide physical rather than chemical protection by preventing light from reaching your skin. Sun blocks do not have SPF ratings. They are good protection for your lips, nose and other particularly sensitive areas, but because they are messy and cover like paint, they are rarely used on large areas.

and give you extra energy. A tiny gland located at the base of your brain, the pineal gland, has been found to secrete a hormone called melatonin during periods of darkness. The gland's secretion of melatonin is suppressed in the presence of bright sunlight.

Melatonin can have adverse emotional, physical and mental effects, according to recent studies. Sunlight can suppress melatonin's depressive effects: Standard indoor lighting is not strong enough to accomplish this. Melatonin can disturb your sleep, bring on feelings of sadness, increase appetite, agitation, fatigue and decrease your efficiency at whatever you do. These symptoms have been reported in people who suffer serious wintertime depressions, an affliction aptly named SAD, for seasonal affective disorder. SAD sufferers usually cheer up in the spring, with the coming of longer, lighter days. Winter vacations in tropical climates can be a more immediate antidote for people who have this disorder. Just be sure to pack plenty of sunscreen.

Traveling

Travelers are faced with a variety of special concerns: Their regular dietary habits are disrupted and normal routines of activity and sleep are altered. Furthermore, travelers may not have access to their usual network of health resources. Thus, even small illnesses can become more serious. But most health problems can be avoided or minimized by a little common sense and advance planning.

If you are going abroad, review your medical records and insurance coverage before your trip. If you have not had recent medical and dental checkups, see your doctor and dentist before you leave. Pregnant women, people taking prescription medications regularly, those recovering from illnesses and individuals with chronic health problems should discuss their travel plans with a doctor. If you become ill or have an accident abroad, contact the nearest United States embassy or consulate, which should refer you to reliable medical care.

It is wise to carry a written summary of your health history: immunization records, lists of your medications by brands and generic names, doctors' letters about your medical problems, a copy of your latest ECG (if you are a heart patient), lists of any drug allergies, and your doctors' telephone numbers. People with serious allergies or special conditions, such as epilepsy or diabetes, should wear identification bracelets indicating the diagnoses and medical precautions.

Find out whether your regular medical insurance will cover illnesses and hospitalizations abroad. Many policies, including Medicare, will not pay for medical problems that occur in other countries. Blue Cross/Blue Shield is recognized worldwide, but most hospitals abroad will not bill Blue Cross, so you will have to pay cash; you will need receipts for reimbursement. If you decide to get additional coverage for a long or hazardous trip, consult the latest edition of Health Information for International Travel, which can be acquired through the Government Printing Office in Washington, DC. Credit-card companies also offer medical insurance abroad.

If you are traveling in underdeveloped regions, make sure to get proper immunization. Check with your doctor or local health department, or consult Health Information for International Travel, which lists immunization requirements for all countries. Since some immunizations require a series of shots, and some may counteract the effects of others, arrange to get them at least six weeks before your trip. Even if you are not traveling in Third World countries, be sure that your tetanus and polio boosters are recent.

Coping with Air Travel

Most long-distance travel begins with an airplane flight, a point at which many traveling problems first arise. Jet lag is one of the most common complaints of air travelers. The box (*opposite*) gives some tips for avoiding jet lag.

Air quality is another concern of some jet travelers. Indeed, while air quality is regulated in airport buildings, federal regulations do not apply to the interiors of planes. Ventilation in airplane cabins is poor, and carbon monoxide levels are high.

The main contaminant of cabin air is cigarette smoke, which can reach extremely high concentrations, even in nonsmoking sections. Smoking, however, is now banned on domestic flights that last less than two hours. And some major carriers, such as Air Canada and Northwest Airlines, have smoke-free flights.

In addition, relative humidity is in the 5- to 10-percent range, which is equivalent to a desert climate that can cause dryness in your eyes, mouth and throat as well as dehydration. It is important, therefore, to drink plenty of fluids, particularly on long flights. But avoid drinks containing alcohol and caffeine, which dehydrate you.

How can you get the best air quality in a plane? If you can afford the fare, choose first class, where ventilation is significantly better than in coach. And if possible, pick flights with smaller, older aircraft. The newer, wide-body planes generally have the poorest ventilation.

Avoiding Infectious Diseases

Even if you have protected youself with immunizations, once you set foot in a foreign country, you must take extra precautions against infectious diseases. To minimize any possibility of becoming infected with the AIDS virus, avoid hypodermics and other medical equipment that may have been used before and that may not have been properly sterilized. Do not get a tattoo, have your ears pierced or undergo acupuncture when traveling. Unless you are in a life-or-death situation, refuse blood transfusions, blood products, injec-

Overcoming Jet Lag

Fatigue, insomnia, and general malaise are common problems that may affect anyone who crosses more than three time zones in a flight. Jet lag is caused by a disruption of sleep/wake patterns: your biological clock is thrown out of sync. Flying westward lengthens your day, and flying eastward shortens it. Because it compresses the day/night cycle, the eastward flight is most likely to produce jet lag.

◆ One preventive measure is to start shifting your sleep/wake cycle to the new time in advance. If traveling east to west, go to bed — and get up — an hour later each day for three days before departure. For a west-to-east trip, move your sleep time an hour earlier each day. If traveling great distances, schedule a stopover if you can.

◆ The jet-lag diet may also be a helpful measure to take. The principle behind this diet is to eat high-protein meals when you are trying to stay awake and high-carbohydrate meals when you want to sleep. A study of U.S. military travelers found that this system alleviated jet lag. Start this diet three days before departure, alternating feast days comprised of high-protein breakfast and lunch and a high-carbohydrate dinner with fast days made up of salads, soup and fruits in small quantities. If you do not want to upset your dietary habits in this manner, you may do as well by getting plenty of rest before the trip and by assuming local eating and sleeping times as soon as you arrive.

◆ Studies show that once you arrive at your destination, you can most quickly reset your biological clock and overcome jet lag by staying in the sun as much as possible. Using this method, most people can become fully acclimated to local time within two days, rather than a week or so had they stayed indoors.

tions, immunizations and vaccinations when traveling in underdeveloped regions. And wherever you are, remember that casual sex can be dangerous. If you take a new sexual partner, always be sure to practice safe sex. See pages 112-113 for information on safe sex.

Food Contamination

Generally, the water and food are safe in Europe, Canada, Japan, Australia and New Zealand. Elsewhere, and even in some rural areas of southern Europe, contaminated water and food can cause traveler's diarrhea as well as serious diseases such as cholera and hepatitis.

When you are away from well-traveled areas, do not drink hotel or restaurant water, brush your teeth with it, eat raw foods that were washed in it or use ice cubes that may have been made from it. Purify water in one of two ways: Boil it for 10 to 15 minutes or add purifying tablets, such as Halozone. Safe beverages usually include coffee and tea (provided that the water has been boiled), bottled wine and beer, and canned soft drinks.

Vegetables are only safe when cooked, and fresh fruits should only be eaten if they are intact, with no breaks in the skin. Wash them with soap and water, rinse them with boiled water, then peel them. When eating meat and fish dishes, be sure they are cooked thoroughly, and eat them hot. If no refrigeration is available, fish should be prepared, cooked and eaten within two hours of being caught. Otherwise, do not eat it. Do not eat raw shellfish and avoid dairy products entirely if you are unsure of their freshness.

Vitamins and Minerals

Vitamins are probably the most misunderstood substances in the realm of nutrition. There are 13 vitamins, each of which performs specific functions in your body's cells and tissues. A healthy individual who eats a well-balanced diet usually meets the Recommended Dietary Allowances (RDAs) for the vitamins listed below.

About 40 percent of American adults take vitamin supplements, even though no study has ever proved that taking them provides much benefit (pregnant women, alcoholics and people recovering from

Vitamins

ADULT RDA*	MAIN FUNCTIONS	SOURCES
A 800–1,000 mcg (micrograms)	Promotes good vision; helps form and maintain healthy skin and mucous membranes; builds bones and teeth; necessary for reproduction; may protect against cancer	Fortified milk and margarine, cheese, eggs, liver, carrots, sweet potatoes, spinach, broccoli, apricots, cantaloupe
C 60 mg (milligrams)	Aids in healing; promotes healthy capillaries, teeth and gums; increases resistance; aids in iron absorption; maintains connective tissue; may block nitrosamines	Citrus fruit, melon, strawberries, potatoes, tomatoes, green peppers, dark green vegetables
D 5–10 mcg	Promotes strong bones and teeth; aids in absorption of calcium and phosphorus	Fortified milk, fish, egg yolks; also produced by your body in response to sunlight
E 8–10 mg	Important for red blood cells; protects tissue against oxidation; helps your body use vitamin K	Nuts, seeds, wheat germ, whole grains, vegetable oils, green leafy vegetables, margarine
K 70–140 mcg**	Aids in blood clotting	Your body produces half its daily needs; beef liver, milk, cauliflower, cabbage, spinach, broccoli
B₁ (thiamin) 1–1.5 mg	Aids in energy release from carbohydrates; necessary for healthy brain and nerve cells and for heart function	Pork, whole grains, dried beans, nuts
B₂ (riboflavin) 1.2–1.7 mg	Aids in energy release from foods; interacts and combines with other B vitamins	Dairy products, liver, whole grains, dark green leafy vegetables, nuts
B₃ (niacin) 13–19 mg	Aids in energy release from foods; synthesis of DNA; maintains functioning of skin, nerves and digestive system	Dairy products, eggs, meat, fish, whole grains, nuts, dried beans and peas
B₅ (pantothenic acid) 4–7 mg**	Aids in energy release from foods; essential for synthesis of numerous body materials	Eggs, whole grains, dried beans, nuts
B₆ (pyridoxine) 2–2.2 mg	Important in chemical reactions of proteins and amino acids; involved in brain function and formation of red blood cells	Fish, meat, whole grains, green leafy vegetables, nuts, bananas
B₁₂ (cobalamin) 3 mcg	Necessary for red blood cells; maintains normal functioning of nervous system	Liver, beef, shellfish, eggs, milk
Folacin (folic acid) 400 mcg	Important in the synthesis of DNA; necessary for cell division and cell immunity	Liver, wheat bran, green leafy vegetables, dried beans and peas, grains
Biotin 100–200 mcg**	Essential for fatty acids; helps metabolize amino acids and carbohydrates	Yeast, liver, eggs, milk

*These figures are not applicable to pregnant or lactating women, who need additional vitamins.
**Although there is no RDA for this vitamin, the Food and Nutrition Board of the National Academy of Sciences recommends this intake range.

surgery or with some other medical condition may require supplements). It is important to remember that supplements can neither be taken in lieu of food nor turn a junk-food diet into a healthy one. Vitamins only work with other nutrients that are present in your diet. See pages 104-105 for information about maintaining a balanced diet.

Minerals are also essential to numerous vital processes in your body. However, minerals consumed in amounts greater than the RDAs or estimated safe intakes may cause serious harm.

Because of the dangers of taking overdoses, you should not self-prescribe mineral supplements. The best way to ensure getting an adequate supply of minerals is to eat a balanced diet. If you believe that you have a mineral deficiency, consult your physician.

Minerals

ADULT RDA*	MAIN FUNCTIONS	SOURCES
Calcium *800 mg* (1,200-1,500 mg for older women)*	Important for healthy bones, teeth, heartbeat, blood clotting and muscle contraction; may help prevent hypertension	Milk products, sardines (with bones), oysters, kale, broccoli, bean curd (tofu)
Chloride *1,700-5,100 mg***	Maintains fluid balance, blood pH; forms hydrochloric acid in the stomach	Fish, table salt, pickled and smoked foods
Chromium *.05-.20 mg***	Important for glucose metabolism; may help control blood glucose concentration	Cheese, meats, whole grains, dried peas and beans, brewer's yeast, peanuts
Copper *2-3 mg***	Formation of red blood cells; necessary for absorption of iron; production of respiration enzymes; interacts with zinc	Shellfish (especially oysters), pork and beef liver, dried beans, chocolate, raisins, nuts, margarine
Fluorine (fluoride) *1.5-4.0 mg***	Aids in the formation of strong bones and teeth; helps prevent cavities in children	Fluoridated water (also foods grown or cooked with it), seafood, tea, gelatin
Iodine *.15 mg**	Necessary for function of thyroid gland and cells; keeps skin, hair and nails healthy; prevents goiter	Iodized salt, seafood, seaweed, vegetables grown in iodine-rich areas, vegetable oil
Iron *10 mg (women over 50 and all men) 18 mg (women 11-50)**	Essential for hemoglobin, which carries oxygen in the blood; forms various enzymes that help fight infection	Red meat, liver (especially pork liver), egg yolks, peas, beans, nuts, dried fruits, green leafy vegetables, enriched grain products, blackstrap molasses
Magnesium *300 mg (women)* 350 mg (men)*	Builds bones; aids function of nerves and muscles, including regulation of heartbeat	Wheat bran, whole grains, raw green leafy vegetables, soybeans, nuts, bananas, apricots, hard water
Manganese *2.5-5.0 mg***	Required for bones, reproduction and cell function	Egg yolks, instant coffee, tea, fruits, vegetables, whole grains, nuts, beans, cocoa powder
Molybdenum *.15-.50 mg***	Important for cell function	Organ meats, peas, beans, cereal grains, dark green vegetables
Phosphorus *800 mg**	Strengthens bones and teeth; important in the metabolism of energy	Fish, poultry, meat, cheese, egg yolks, milk products, dried peas and beans, soft drinks
Potassium *1,875-5,625 mg***	Promotes regular heartbeat; aids in muscle contraction; regulates transfer of nutrients; controls water balance	Bananas, oranges, peanut butter, dried peas and beans, meat, potatoes, coffee, tea, cocoa, yogurt, molasses
Selenium *05-.20 mg***	Works with vitamin E to fight cell damage by oxygen; necessary for immunity enzymes and antibodies	Seafood, red meat, egg yolks, chicken, garlic, milk
Sodium *1,100-3,300 mg***	Helps regulate water balance in body; aids in maintaining blood pressure	Salt, high-sodium processed foods
Zinc *15 mg**	Necessary for growth, sexual and fetal development and healing; part of enzymes necessary for immune cells	Oysters, crabmeat, beef, liver, poultry, eggs, brewer's yeast, whole grains

Weight Control

There is no single, authoritative formula for determining your ideal weight. A simple technique for estimating whether you are heavier than you should be is the pinch test. Hold up one arm as if you were going to flex your muscle (but do not actually flex it). With the thumb and forefinger of your other hand, gently pinch the skin on the back of your arm, just below your triceps muscle. Release the skin and measure the space between your thumb and forefinger. If it is greater than an inch, you should consider reducing your body weight.

Body weight is an integral part of a person's self-image. And Americans, in particular, are preoccupied with gaining and losing weight. The ideal body proportions are often depicted as lean and trim, yet many people are overweight. A report from the National Institutes of Health estimated that 34 million adult Americans weigh more than they should, according to average height and weight standards.

What motivates most people to control their weight is concern about their appearance. When you gain weight — or lose it — people notice. However, if you are more than a few pounds overweight, there are also compelling benefits to be gained from losing fat.

As excess weight increases, so do health risks. Many long-term studies have established that high-fat diets, which often lead to weight gain, are associated with increased risk for a range of diseases, including hypertension, diabetes, stroke, certain types of cancer, and high cholesterol levels and heart attacks. One major study indicated that for every 10 percent weight reduction in men aged 35 to 55, there is a 20 percent decrease in coronary heart disease. Extra pounds can also place increased stress on your bones and ligaments; the burden can be especially great on your back, since weight often settles around your abdomen, pulling your spine forward.

Many health-care professionals think that, of all the adverse effects of being overweight, the greatest is the psychological stress that often accompanies weight gain. There is a social stigma attached to being heavier than average standards, perhaps borne by a common assumption that visible fat is a sign of being weak-willed and self-indulgent. In many instances, losing weight can make an important difference in your self-image and how others see you.

Why some people are overweight and others stay thin easily has not been fully answered. Genetic factors and aging certainly affect body weight: Most people tend to gain weight as they get older, possibly because of a drop in basal metabolism. They may metabolize food at a slower rate; unless they eat less, calories are converted into body fat. Also, many people become less active.

Some researchers have speculated that your body weight has a "set point," which is a precise amount of fat that it strives to maintain. There is also some evidence that people prone to obesity burn calories at a lower rate than others, even when their activity level is the same.

Nevertheless, most researchers agree that lifestyle and eating habits are major factors that affect your weight. Modifying these factors is the key to weight control for most people, particularly those who diet repeatedly, only to regain the weight that was lost at a previous time. Basically, when you eat foods that contain more energy, which is measured in calories, than your body expends in daily activities, the excess calories are stored as body fat. To lose weight, you need to consume less food and increase your physical activity until your energy output exceeds your caloric intake.

Losing weight has two phases: reducing pounds and keeping the weight off by adopting changes in your diet and exercise habits on a long-term basis. Most diet plans emphasize only the first phase, which is

Tactics for Cutting Calories

◆ Eating less fat is the most efficient way of cutting your caloric intake. Ounce for ounce, fat has more than twice the calories of protein and carbohydrates. This means limiting your intake of butter, whole milk, cheese, ice cream, salad dressing and oil. Also, avoid packaged snacks, cookies, and baked goods — such foods are usually high in fat.

◆ Replace high-fat foods with foods rich in complex carbohydrates — cereals, grains, legumes and vegetables. One university study showed that obese subjects consumed about 1,600 calories a day when their foods were high in complex carbohydrates; when the foods were low in complex carbohydrates but high in fat, they consumed approximately 3,000 calories a day.

◆ Include only the leanest cuts of meat in your diet several times a week in small portions (three to four ounces). Better yet, eat lean fish or white-meat poultry. Bake, broil or poach meats and steam vegetables (rather than fry or sauté them in fat).

◆ Change your eating habits: Use smaller dishes to make portions seems bigger; chew slowly and put your utensils down between mouthfuls; leave the table immediately after eating; pause in the middle of each meal. In regard to exercise, increase your routine daily activity through walking and climbing stairs; and gradually start a regular program of aerobic exercise such as running, cycling or rowing.

easier to accomplish than a permanent change in lifestyle. And most of these diets make claims to provide quick weight loss with particular food combinations, special meal schedules or dramatic reductions in calories. Unfortunately, many people who rely on these quick-remedy diets regain the weight they lost within one or two years after the diet.

Nutritionists recommend weight-loss programs that contain a moderate amount of calories, resulting in an energy deficit of about 500 calories per day. For most people, it means consuming no fewer than 1,200 calories per day. This will not produce quick weight losses, but most experts agree that you should try to lose no more than two pounds per week. Moreover, a balanced diet provides the only nutritionally sound basis for maintaining weight loss.

The other element of an effective weight-control program is exercise. A number of studies indicate that many obese people do not gorge themselves with food; they are simply more sedentary than people of average weight. Other studies show that adults who stay physically active are also better able to maintain their normal weight. The chief benefit of combining exercise with a proper low-calorie diet is that it helps maintain lean body mass — muscle and organ tissue.

To keep your body at its optimal weight, take a gradual approach in your eating plan and exercise habits. If you cut out 200 to 300 calories per day — the equivalent of a serving of mayonnaise on a sandwich — and exercise vigorously for 15 minutes daily, you will lose approximately a pound of body fat in less than two weeks. Healthy lifestyle changes that are made slowly are easier to incorporate into your daily routine. However you structure your diet and exercise program, you should lose about one to one and a half pounds per week. See the box (above) for other tips.

Medical Self-Tests

In addition to regular examinations and proper medical care, self-exams and self-diagnostic tests can help you guard against poor health and provide you with a heightened sense of control over your body. However, they should never be used as a replacement for a physician and regular medical checkups.

Self-tests can be conducted by people who know or suspect that they have a particular medical condition. Self-exams can be especially valuable in discovering the early symptoms of skin, breast and testicular cancer. Popular self-test kits are explained on this and the facing page and self-examinations are explained on pages 134-135.

If you find a suspicious growth, lesion or any other abnormality when you perform a self-exam, or get a positive result on a self-test, seek medical attention immediately. Most conditions, when caught early, can be treated effectively. Keep in mind that positive results on tests do not necessarily mean that you have various conditions; a physician will conduct further investigations to verify the self-test's outcome. In addition, negative results are not substitutes for regular medical checkups.

Self-Test Kits

BLOOD GLUCOSE MONITORING

Purpose: Measures the concentration of blood glucose, which reflects the body's ability to use carbohydrates. This test is useful for diabetics, who adjust their diet and insulin doses to meet their daily needs. Well-controlled blood glucose may reduce the major complications of diabetes—nerve damage, kidney and heart disease and blindness. Perform the test under a physician's supervision.

Procedure: With clean and dry hands, a drop of blood is obtained by pricking a fingertip. The blood is then placed on a chemically treated test strip, which changes color when it reacts with blood glucose. After waiting the specified time, the blood is lightly wiped off the test strip. After another time period, results are determined by matching the color on the test strip to a color chart included in the kit. The blood glucose concentration will influence the color intensity. Test strips can also be used with an electronic glucose meter. These portable meters show the blood glucose level on a digital display and are usually equipped with built-in timers that pace each step. Blood glucose monitoring is more accurate than testing urine for glucose content. *Time for results: one to two minutes*

Comments: Electronic glucose meters are simpler to read and more precise than the color strips. If the results are surprising or questionable, repeat the test. If results are inconsistent with bodily symptoms, consult your doctor.

BLOOD PRESSURE MONITORING

Purpose: Monitors blood pressure at home. For hypertensives, frequent monitoring of blood pressure can provide a better understanding of blood pressure patterns, which are affected by various activities, diet and medications.

Procedure: Most blood pressure-measuring kits contain a sphygmomanometer (measuring device), a cuff or air bladder, and either a stethoscope or a microphone. Place the center of the cuff (or microphone) directly on the pulse point located in the artery of the upper arm. Wrap the cuff snugly around the upper arm and quickly inflate it until it cuts off the blood flow—until about 30 mm/Hg higher than your usual systolic pressure, or to 210 mm/Hg. Blood pressure readings are obtained by releasing the pressure and listening for the arterial pulsations. *Time for results: two to five minutes*

Comments: To find out what your readings mean, check the blood pressure classifications on page 34. Repeated measurements are important since a single reading may be inaccurate. To improve accuracy, take the average of three readings, five to ten minutes apart. If your average blood pressure is above 140/90 mm/Hg, consult your doctor. Never change or discontinue blood pressure medication without your doctor's instructions. Be certain to take your pressure at the same time each day and under the same conditions. Factors that can cause fluctuations in test results include: smoking, exercising, eating or drinking just prior to the test, noise, stress, medications, moving during the test and cuffs that are not positioned or used properly. Make sure the cuff is the right size. Check the accuracy of your device against readings obtained by a health professional with a mercury column device.

FECAL-OCCULT BLOOD TEST

Purpose: Detects hidden, or occult, blood in stool specimens, which may be a sign of gastrointestinal bleeding, rectal or colon cancer, ulcers, colitis polyps, diverticulitis, hemorrhoids or bleeding gums. These tests should be used only to screen people without symptoms–those who already have visible signs of blood in their stools should consult a physician immediately.

Procedure: Stool specimens are mixed with a chemical solution, which causes color changes to appear if blood is present. The American Cancer Society has recommended that specimens be collected from three consecutive bowel movements. To improve accuracy, certain diet restrictions should be followed two days prior to the test, and until all stool samples are collected. Avoid taking the test if you are bleeding–for example, from body cuts, hemorrhoids or during menstruation. *Time for results: one-half to 16 minutes*

Comments: Consult a doctor immediately if test results are positive. The following factors may cause false-positive results: red meat, radishes, horseradish, turnips, broccoli, cauliflower and melons; iron supplements and certain medications, including aspirin and anti-inflammatory drugs. Factors that may cause false-negative results include: taking vitamin C supplements or laxatives containing mineral oil. If the test results are negative, but symptoms such as unusual weight loss or changes in bowel habits persist for more than two weeks, consult a doctor.

OVULATION MONITORING

Purpose: Detects changes in the amount of luteinizing hormone (LH) in the urine and can be used to calculate when a woman is most fertile. LH is secreted during the menstrual cycle, but at the middle of it, there is a sudden increase in LH, known as the LH surge, which indicates ovulation. Ovulation usually occurs 24 to 36 hours after the beginning of the LH surge.

Procedure: Midway between menstrual periods, dip a test strip into the first morning urine sample daily for approximately one week. An LH surge is detected by matching color changes on the test strip with a color chart. *Time for results: 20 minutes to one hour*

Comments: Not a reliable form of contraception. Consult your doctor immediately if there is an LH surge for more than four consecutive days.

PREGNANCY TESTS

Purpose: Tests the urine for the presence of the human chorionic gonadotropin (HCG) hormone, which is produced during pregnancy by the developing placenta.

Procedure: Tests are performed in a test tube or with a chemically treated test strip. Collect the first morning urine specimen. A positive result is indicated by a color change on a test strip or in the solution, or by the presence of a ring-shaped deposit, which can be seen at the bottom of a test tube. Perform it at least seven to nine days after an expected menstrual period does not occur. Some physicians recommend waiting at least 14 days for the tube-type tests. *Time for results: 20 minutes to two hours*

Comments: If the test is positive, see your physician to confirm the results. If the result is negative, there is still a possibility that you are pregnant. Repeat the test about one week after the negative result if your period has not occurred. After two negative test results, consult your physician if you are still not menstruating.

URINARY-TRACT INFECTIONS

Purpose: Detects the presence of nitrite in urine. Gram-negative bacteria, which are responsible for most urinary-tract infections, convert digested dietary nitrate into nitrite.

Procedure: Nitrite is detected by dipping a chemically treated test strip into a urine sample on three consecutive mornings. If there is a uniform color change, nitrite is present, indicating that bacteria are present in the urinary tract. *Time for results: 30 to 40 seconds*

Comments: Notify your physician immediately if you obtain positive results. Since the tests do not detect gram-positive bacteria, which are responsible for 10 percent of infections, false-negative results are possible. High doses of vitamin C and testing a urine sample that was not in the bladder for at least four hours can also cause false-negative results. If your result is negative, but symptoms persist, such as itching or burning with frequent urination or the presence of discharge, consult your physician.

Skin Examination

The skin, the largest organ, is more prone to develop cancer than any other part of the body. The best way to locate a potentially cancerous area of skin is by performing a monthly skin check as described below. You need a full-length mirror, a hand-held mirror, a blow dryer and two chairs. If you find a suspicious sign, contact a physician immediately. While most skin cancers are curable, it is essential that they be detected and treated early. Even malignant melanoma, the most serious and life-threatening form of skin cancer, can often be successfully treated and cured when it is detected early.

THREE TYPES OF SKIN CANCER

Basal-cell carcinoma	Squamous-cell carcinoma	Malignant melanoma
Raised and translucent nodules often located on the hands, neck, head and torso that often bleed, crust and open up again. This is the most common form of skin cancer; usually not life-threatening, but can destroy underlying tissue. It does not metastasize.	Appears as a reddish nodule, patch or warty growth often located on the face, ears or hands. It may increase in size, bleed or ulcerate. If left untreated, it can metastasize to other body parts, causing serious damage and death.	Begins as a large, irregular and/or multishaded mole or lesion. This is the most dangerous and least common form of skin cancer. It can metastasize throughout the body, if left undiagnosed and untreated, and eventually cause death.

What to Look For: Sores that do not heal • Moles that exceed size of a pencil eraser • Asymmetrical moles with irregular borders • Moles or blemishes that appear mottled or have various shades and colors • Sores that scale, crust, soften, ooze, bleed or produce nodules • Moles or blemishes that hurt, itch or are increasingly sensitive

How to Perform the Self-Exam:

1 After bathing or showering, stand in a well-lighted room in front of a full-length mirror. Examine the fronts, backs and sides of your hands, fingers and fingernails. Check your armpits, elbows and the fronts and backs of your forearms and upper arms. Use the full-length mirror and hand mirror to provide complete views of each area that you inspect.

2 With both mirrors, examine your face and neck, which both are common areas of cancerous skin growths. Then closely check your shoulders, chest and abdomen.

3 Examine the back of your neck and your back. Then check your buttocks, the backs of your thighs and your lower legs.

4 Set your blow dryer on a low speed and temperature. Hold it in one hand and the mirror in the other. Examine your scalp by blowing hair upward to allow maximum visibility.

5 Sit down on one chair and prop one leg up on the second chair. With your hand mirror, closely examine the bottoms of your feet, your toes, toenails and the spaces between your toes. Moving upward, check the tops of your feet, ankles, calves, thighs and groin.

Breast Examination

It is important for women to perform monthly breast exams. Men should perform the same procedure, since breast cancer is a risk for men as well. Menstruating women should examine their breasts regularly a few days after their periods end. Women who are no longer menstruating, and all men, should choose one day in the month to perform their self-exams. If you discover a change in your breast tissue, make an appointment to see your doctor immediately. Do not be frightened; most lumps and changes in your breasts are not cancerous. However, if breast cancer is diagnosed, it is often curable when detected and treated in the early stages. In addition to monthly self-exams, women between 18 and 40 should have their breasts examined by a physician every three years; those over the age of 40 should be examined annually. You should also have a baseline mammogram performed at age 35 followed by regular mammograms every one to two years after age 40 and annual mammograms after age 50.

What to Look For: Changes from previous exams ● Lumps or thickened areas ● Redness, swelling, puckering and scaling of skin or sores ● Discharge from nipples and changes in direction

---

How to Perform the Self-Exam:

1 Stand in front of a mirror and examine your breasts for changes in size and shape. Check for dimpling, puckering and scaling of the skin. Relax your arms at your sides, then raise them and clasp your hands behind your head. Place your hands on your hips and bend your elbows forward. Using your thumb and index finger, gently squeeze each nipple and examine for discharge.

2 *Because your fingers move easily over wet, soapy skin, perform the following exam in the shower or bath.*
Raise your right arm and position your hand behind your head. Use the pads of the fingers of your left hand to examine your right breast. With enough pressure to feel the deep tissue, begin at the outer edge, slowly moving your fingers in a circular motion toward the nipple. Continue this exam in your armpit and the side of your breast. Repeat this procedure for your left breast.

3 *While lying down, continue to examine your breasts, feeling for lumps or any tenderness beneath the skin.*
With a pillow placed beneath your right shoulder, raise your right hand and place it behind your head. Using the circular motions described in step 2, examine your right breast. Position a pillow beneath your left shoulder and repeat for your left breast.

Testicular Examination

Testicular cancer usually strikes men between the ages of 15 and 35. It is responsible for approximately 12 percent of all cancer deaths in this age group, and it is the number-one cause of cancer fatalities among men in their twenties and thirties. As with most cancers, early detection and treatment is crucial. The American Cancer Society recommends the following monthly self-exam. If you discover any irregularity while performing it, consult your doctor immediately.

What to Look For: Small, firm, painless lumps attached to the testicles ● Slight swelling in one or both testicles ● Change in the consistency of the testicles

---

How to Perform the Self-Exam:
The best time to examine your testes is after a warm shower or bath, when the scrotal skin and muscles are relaxed.

1 In a standing position, check your scrotal sac to be sure that both testicles are properly descended. Although an undescended testicle is fairly common, this condition greatly increases your risk of testicular cancer.

2 While standing, extend your left leg and rest it on a chair. Hold your left testicle with both hands; gently roll it between your thumbs and fingers, feeling for any irregular texture. Place your right leg on a chair and repeat the exam for your right testicle.

3 Examine each testicle for enlargement. It is common for the left testicle to hang somewhat below the right one, but both testicles should be about the same size.

First Aid

A knowledge of first aid can enable you to provide immediate care to someone who is injured or who has suddenly become ill. First aid should be applied whenever medical assistance is delayed or unavailable.

The first step in assisting an injured person is to check his breathing. Then make sure that the victim's heart is beating by checking his pulse. After checking for these vital functions, you should examine him for bleeding. Do not attempt cardiopulmonary resuscitation unless you have received CPR training.

Do not move the victim if there is any possibility of spinal injuries, unless his location poses a serious threat to his safety. Do not give first aid unless you know what you are doing; applying inept care can not only be useless, it can cause more serious injury.

To prepare for the possibility when you may have to use first aid, assemble first-aid kits for your home and auto (see the checklist below). Then familiarize yourself with the techniques shown on the facing page and on pages 138-141. Keep in mind that first-aid procedures can vary or not always apply to people with specific medical conditions, infants, and to those who are pregnant, obese or have spinal, neck or head injuries.

First-Aid Kit

A well-stocked first-aid kit is essential to all households. The following items should be stored in a sturdy box that can be closed securely. Store the kit in a convenient but childproof location; the kitchen is often the best place because it is where many household injuries occur. Remember to restock used items. Store a second first-aid kit in the trunk of your car.

Adhesive tape	Paper cups
Rubbing alcohol	Flashlight with extra batteries
Antibiotic cream	Safety pins
Thermometer	Scissors (blunt ends)
Aspirin	Soap bar, mild
Adhesive bandages, assorted sizes	Sodium bicarbonate (baking soda)

Six elastic roller bandages
  two 1 inch by 5 yards
  two 2 inches by 5 yards
  two 3 inches by 5 yards
	Hydrogen peroxide (3 percent solution)

	Splints, several ¼ inch thick
	  12-15 inches long
	  3½ inches wide
	  several 3-inch finger splints

Calamine lotion	
Sterile cotton balls	Rubber tourniquet several inches wide and about 20 inches long

Sterile first-aid dressings
  one 2 inches square
  one 4 inches square
	Two large towels or sheets*

	Two small towels*
Epsom salts	Tweezers
Instant cold compresses	Pocketknife
Syrup of ipecac	

To avoid risk of infection, always be sure that towels and sheets are clean.

Mouth-to-Mouth Resuscitation

You may encounter someone who needs mouth-to-mouth resuscitation almost anywhere. Pools, lakes and the seashore are common sites because of drowning risks. Electric shocks, burns or poisoning can also cause respiratory arrest. A few common symptoms of someone in need of resuscitation are dilated pupils, pale or blue lips and loss of consciousness. Whatever the cause of respiratory arrest, you must act quickly: Without oxygen, a victim can suffer permanent brain damage or death within approximately six minutes. Read the following procedures carefully.

TREATMENT

1 Roll the person over onto his back. Open the victim's mouth and clear away any objects, such as chewing gum or food, from the mouth and airway.

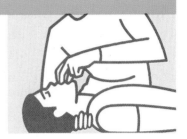

2 If the victim's neck does not appear to be injured, with your hand under his neck, gently lift it upward so his head tilts back. Place your other hand on his forehead and push down to raise his chin upward.

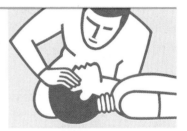

3 With one hand on the victim's forehead, use your thumb and index finger to pinch his nostrils closed. Breathe in deeply, position your mouth snugly around the victim's mouth and exhale. Quickly give him four breaths without permitting his lungs to deflate fully.

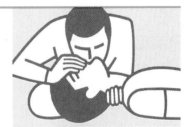

4 When the chest is fully expanded, remove your mouth and place your ear above the victim's mouth so you can hear the air leaving his lungs. Repeat the procedure every five seconds until he begins to breathe without assistance or until medical help arrives.

5 Once the victim's breathing is restored, treat for shock, then seek medical care.

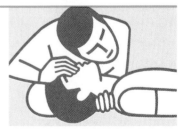

How to Stop Severe Bleeding

Serious bleeding must be stopped. When treating a bleeding victim, remove clothing from the wound area and proceed with the following instructions. After bleeding has stopped or slowed, treat the victim for shock.

DIRECT-PRESSURE TECHNIQUE

- Check the victim's breathing and make sure an open airway is maintained.
- Put a clean cloth over the wound. (If no cloth is available, use your bare hand.)
- With the palm of your hand, apply firm and constant pressure directly on the wound.
- If blood soaks through the compress, do not remove it; place another compress over it.
- Apply pressure more firmly over a larger area.
- If the wound is on the leg, arm, hand or neck, lay the victim down and elevate the area above the victim's heart while applying direct pressure.
- When the bleeding stops or slows, tie a pressure bandage over the compress with gauze or a cloth strip. Place the middle of the bandage over the compress, wrap the ends around the wound and knot it over the compress.
- Keep the affected area elevated above the victim's heart.
- Treat the victim for shock if necessary.
- Phone for medical attention.

PRESSURE-POINT TECHNIQUE

This should only be used if bleeding does not slow or stop after applying direct pressure and elevation. Always use the pressure-point technique in conjunction with direct pressure and elevation. Never use it any longer than absolutely necessary. However, if you stop applying pressure and bleeding begins again, reapply the pressure-point technique.

Bleeding Arms:

- Hold the victim's arm halfway between his elbow and armpit.
- Position your thumb on the outside of his arm and your fingers on the inside.
- Squeeze your thumb and fingers toward each other and against his arm bone until the wound stops bleeding.

Bleeding Legs:

- If possible, position the victim on his back.
- Place the heel of your hand on the crease of his groin, toward the front and center of his thigh.
- Keeping your arm straight, use your body weight to press down so his femoral artery is against his pelvic bone and the bleeding stops.

DO NOT:

- Try to remove or disturb any blood clots on the wound or the compress.
- Elevate the affected area if you suspect a broken bone.
- Remove a compress even if blood soaks through it.
- Wrap a bandage so tightly that it may cut off circulation.
- Use a tourniquet unless you have attempted to control bleeding with other means and the victim is in danger of bleeding to death.

Choking

Choking is a leading cause of accidental death among children and adults. Children may choke on anything they put into their mouths. Adults most often choke when they talk or laugh while eating. When a choking victim's windpipe is fully obstructed, the person will not be able to breathe, cough or speak. A victim will probably appear frantic and may raise one hand toward his throat in a grasping motion. Stay calm and act quickly.

Symptoms of Choking: Person grasps throat • Victim cannot talk • Person gasps for breath and breathes noisily • Victim has difficulty coughing • Breathing stops • Skin turns pale, blue, white or gray • Person exhibits panic in facial expressions and movements • Victim becomes unconscious

TREATMENT

PRELIMINARY ACTION

If Victim is Standing or Sitting:

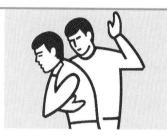

1 Stand behind and somewhat to the side of the victim.

2 Place one hand on his chest for support.

3 Bend him forward.

4 With the heel of your free hand, rapidly and forcefully hit him between the shoulder blades four times.

If Victim is Lying Down:

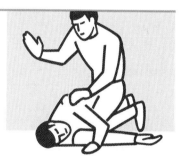

1 Kneel next to him and put your finger in the back of his mouth to clear away food.

2 Roll him onto his side facing you.

3 Press your knees slightly against his chest for support.

4 Using the heel of your hand, hit four powerful blows between his shoulder blades.

If these steps do not restore the victim's ability to breathe, perform the Heimlich maneuver as described below.

HEIMLICH MANEUVER

If Victim is Standing or Sitting:

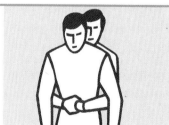

1 Stand or squat behind the choking person.

2 Place both arms around him.

3 Make a fist with one hand and press it against his abdomen, halfway between the bottom of his ribs and navel.

4 With your other hand, grasp your fist and give four fast thrusts in an inward and upward motion with the thumb side of your fist against him.

If Victim is Lying Down:

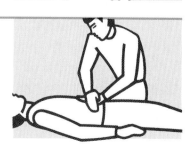

1 Position the person on his back.

2 Kneel beside him.

3 Place the heel of one hand above his navel and below his rib cage.

4 Put your other hand on top of your positioned hand.

5 Quickly and forcefully, give four thrusts downward and toward his head.

If the Heimlich maneuver produces no results, repeat all steps until the object becomes dislodged and the victim is able to cough it up. Stop if the person becomes unconscious. Call for medical assistance immediately.

Burns

Burns are commonly caused by open fires, lit cigarettes, hot liquids, cooking and electrical equipment. The severity of burns is based on how many layers of skin are affected and the body area involved. First-degree burns are the least dangerous and heal quickly. They affect only the outer layer of skin, usually causing pain, slight swelling and redness. Second-degree burns are more painful and affect the layers of skin beneath the surface. Often blisters occur and the affected area remains swollen, blotchy, damp and red for several days. The most serious are third-degree burns, which affect all layers of the skin and underlying tissue. The damaged area may look charred, and there is little pain because the burn has destroyed the nerve endings. Treat a burn victim for the greatest degree of damage suspected. Hospitalization is necessary when burns of any kind cover 15 percent of an adult's body or 10 percent of a child's body.

Get Immediate Medical Attention if the Victim: Has inhaled smoke ● Has burns on his hands, feet or face ● Has extensive first- or second-degree burns ● Has third-degree burns ● Has chemical burns

TREATMENT

If you are in doubt regarding the degree of a burn, treat the area for third-degree burns.

FIRST-DEGREE BURNS:

1 Use a cold-water compress or immerse the burn in cold water for 15 minutes.

2 Pat dry and, if desired, place a clean bandage over the area.

SECOND-DEGREE BURNS:

1 Use a cold-water compress or place the burned area in cold water until pain lessens.

2 Pat dry and cover with a clean cloth or sterile bandage.

3 If feet or legs are burned, raise them; if hands or arms are burned, elevate them above the victim's heart.

THIRD-DEGREE BURNS:

1 If the victim is on fire, use a blanket, rug or coat to put out the flames.

2 Check the victim's breathing. Make sure his airway is open. If he appears to have difficulty breathing, slightly raise his head and shoulders. Perform mouth-to-mouth resuscitation if necessary.

3 Cover burned hands, feet or face with cold cloths or cool water.

4 Place a thick, clean dressing over the burned area. (Sheets, towels or disposable diapers can be used.) If fingers or toes are affected, separate them while bandaging so the skin does not stick together.

5 Cover the victim with a blanket to keep him warm.

6 a) If hands are burned, raise them above the victim's heart.
   b) If feet or legs are burned, elevate them; do not allow the victim to walk.
   c) If neck or face is burned, prop the victim up.

7 Treat the victim for shock if necessary.

8 Call for medical assistance.

CHEMICAL BURNS:

1 Run cold water over the burned area for at least five minutes. Do not use strong pressure.

2 Remove clothing from the affected area while continuing to drench with cold water.

3 If possible, follow the instructions on the label of the substance that has caused the burn.

4 Apply cool, wet compresses to relieve pain.

5 Cover the burned area with a clean dressing.

DO NOT:
Use butter or grease ● Use home remedies, ointments or antiseptics unless recommended by a physician ● Remove clothing or material that appears stuck to the burned area ● Use ice or ice water on any type of burn ● Place cold water on third-degree burns ● Break blisters ● Put pressure on burned areas

---

Poisoning

If you suspect that someone has swallowed a poisonous substance, do not necessarily follow the instructions on labels—they are often outdated and inaccurate. Instead, call a poison-control center, a hospital emergency room or a physician immediately. State what the victim has swallowed, the quantity consumed and how long it will take to transport the victim to a treatment center. Follow instructions given by the poison-control center or your physician. Before emergency assistance arrives, or if it is unavailable, follow the advice below.

IF VICTIM IS UNCONSCIOUS, NOT BREATHING OR HAVING CONVULSIONS:

- Make sure his airway is open.
- If necessary, perform mouth-to-mouth resuscitation.
- Loosen clothing, especially around his waist and neck.
- If he vomits, turn his head to the side to prevent choking.
- If you must move him, place him on his stomach or side with his head turned sideways.
- Collect a sample of vomit to bring to the hospital along with the container of poison.

IF VICTIM IS CONSCIOUS:

- Give the victim at least eight ounces of water or milk to dilute the poison.
- Give only water if he has ingested a gasoline product.
- If he vomits, bend him over so that his head is face down below his waist to prevent choking. If the victim is a small child, position him face down across your knees.

IF INSTRUCTED BY A MEDICAL AUTHORITY, INDUCE VOMITING:

- If the victim is over 12, give him two tablespoons of syrup of ipecac and eight to 16 ounces of milk or water, depending on the poison, as the doctor directs.
- If he is between one and 12, give one tablespoon of syrup of ipecac; give children under five 8 ounces of milk or water.
- If he is under one, give him two teaspoons of syrup of ipecac.
- Vomiting should occur within approximately 20 minutes. If it does not occur, give him one additional dose of syrup of ipecac.
- If no syrup of ipecac is available, tickle the back of his throat with your finger or a spoon.

DO NOT INDUCE VOMITING IF:
- He is unconscious.
- He is having convulsions.
- You do not know what poison he swallowed.
- The poison is a petroleum product such as gasoline, lighter fluid or paint thinner.
- The poison is an acid liquid or substance such as bleach, rust remover or detergent.
- The poison is an alkali liquid or substance such as lye and drain and oven cleaners.

DO NOT GIVE LIQUIDS IF:
- He is unconscious.
- He is having convulsions.

DO NOT:
- Give fruit juice, carbonated drinks, alcohol or vinegar to neutralize the poison.
- Follow the antidote instructions on the label of the poison, especially if it is old; instructions may be incorrect and outdated.
- Give salt or mustard to induce vomiting.

INDEX

PROP CREDITS

Pages 6-7: leotard and leggings–Hind Performance Sportswear, San Luis Obispo, Calif., shoes and socks–Nike, Inc., Beaverton, Ore., rug–ABC International Design Rugs, New York City; pages 22-23: sphygmomanometer–Hammacher Schlemmer, New York City; pages 44-45: shoes–Nike, Inc., Beaverton, Ore.

ACKNOWLEDGMENTS

"Your Medical Age" was adapted from "Medical vs. Current Age Score Card" and reprinted with permission of Grosset & Dunlap from *HOW TO BE YOUR OWN DOCTOR (SOMETIMES)*, copyright 1975, 1981 by Keith W. Sehnert and Howard Eisenberg

All cosmetics and grooming products supplied by Clinique Labs, Inc., New York City.

Nutrition analysis provided by Hill Nutrition Associates, Fayetteville, N.Y.

Index prepared by Carney W. Mimms III

Production by Giga Communications

Photo stylists: cover, pages 6-7, 44-45: Nola Lopez; pages 22-23: Betty Blau

PHOTOGRAPHY CREDITS

Cover, pages 6-7, 22-23, 44-45: Andrew Eccles; title page copyright David Madison

ILLUSTRATION CREDITS

Pages 20-21, 37, 39, 59, 61, 95, 109: David Flaherty; page 26: Brian Sisco; pages 41, 43, 56-57, 69: Dana Burns-Pizer; pages 51, 55, 72, 88-89: Phil Scheuer; pages 91, 137, 139: Tami Colichio; all charts by Brian Sisco